Crisis Management Leadership In The Operating Room –

Prepare Your Team to Survive Any Crisis

Kenneth A. Lipshy, M.D., F.A.C.S.

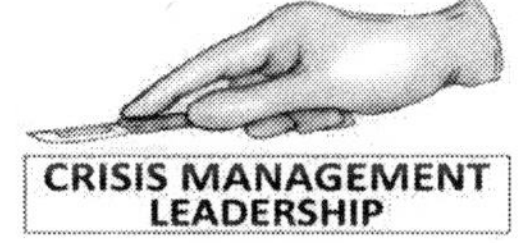

www.CrisisManagementLeadership.com

Creative Team Publishing
San Diego

Disclaimer: The opinions and conclusions expressed in this book are strictly those of the author and do not necessarily represent or express the policies and procedures of the U.S. Department of Defense or the U.S. Department of Veterans Affairs.

ISBN: 978-0-9897975-4-2

PUBLISHED BY CREATIVE TEAM PUBLISHING
www.CreativeTeamPublishing.com
San Diego

Printed in the United States of America

Important Questions
Have you ever…

- Done or witnessed someone doing something that was just plain *stupid?*
- Wondered, "How did we *not see that coming?"*
- Been or witnessed someone or a team who was obviously *in over their head* after a surprise event?
- Viewed a response to an unexpected event as *dysfunctional?*
- Wondered, "How on earth did he, she, or they *survive* that?" Was it luck or planning?

If these questions resonate with you, then this book will be of great interest.

- The question never is whether a crisis is coming.
- The question always is how prepared anyone or any team is to deal with it.
- Handling and managing a crisis requires knowledge and preparation.
- Without either, a crisis can overtake you, and disaster results.
- When knowledge and preparation are part of the training and character of an organization, its leaders

and teams can manage to mitigate crises of almost any magnitude.

- Standard crisis checklists help organize a functional team, but only if they are trained to survive the initial stages of the crisis and can become organized.

The uniqueness of this book is its firsthand instructions from military and first responders as to how any organization--your organization--should respond in crisis. The question isn't whether or not a crisis is potentially possible; the real question for the high-risk professional is always, *"Are we appropriately prepared to respond to this crisis?"*

If you want the answers to those questions from the people who live and work in crisis-driven situations on a recurring basis, read on. If you are a member of an Operating Room Team you already know this strikes to the heart of who you are and what you do. Indeed, this may be the most important work on management leadership in a crisis that you have ever read.

Be prepared... *you never know when your preparation can save the lives of others as well as your own.*

Crisis Management Leadership In The Operating Room –

Prepare Your Team to Survive Any Crisis

Kenneth A. Lipshy, M.D., F.A.C.S.

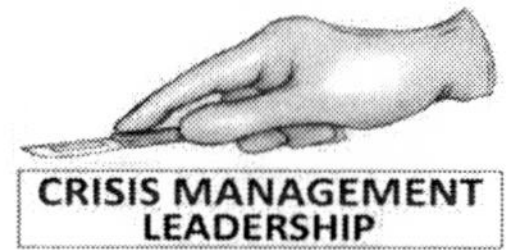

Endorsements on Behalf of *Crisis Management Leadership In The Operating Room*

George C. Velmahos, MD, PhD, MSEd ,
John F. Burke Professor of Surgery,
Harvard Medical School, Chief – Division of Trauma,
Emergency Surgery, and Surgical Critical Care,
Massachusetts General Hospital

This book is invaluable not only for its content but also for the way it passes the information. In a technically masterful fashion Dr. Lipshy uses a direct style of language, representative figures and diagrams, and appropriate evidence to make the text flow naturally and easy to read.

The case about cohesive team building and leadership through crisis is made effectively, and practical solutions are given. I must admit that the book was an eye-opener to me in so many ways.
~ George C. Velmahos

*****

John A. Weigelt, MD, DVM, MMA
Department of Surgery, Trauma Division/
CC Medical College of Wisconsin
Milt and Lidy Lunda Aprahamian
Professor of Surgery,
Associate Dean of Clinical Quality,
Medical College of Wisconsin
Editor in Chief, *Journal of Surgical Education*

Healthcare providers are constantly being told that we need to improve safety within our healthcare system. Multiple suggestions are made regarding how to achieve a safer environment, but are these principles of a highly reliable organization reaching the front lines of surgical practice? Dr. Lipshy has taken many of the basic principles of safety, teamwork, performance improvement, and crisis management and put them together for the operating room environment.

This book helps us understand how problems occur in the operating room. It suggests how methods from other disciplines can be used to control, mitigate, and possibly avoid these crisis situations. The book is well written. Its scenarios will be readily recognized by surgeons and anesthesiologists. Given the emphasis on safety and quality within our training programs, I suggest it might even appear on a required reading list for surgical trainees and teams.
~ John A. Weigelt

Jeffrey S. Young, MD, MBA, Professor of Surgery,
Director, Trauma Center, and
Chief Patient Safety Officer,
University of Virginia Health System

Patient care at the bedside has been neglected in the patient safety revolution in favor of metrics and colored dots. This book tries to bring this imbalance back into equilibrium. It is the critical decisions and teamwork around the operating table that save lives during unexpected events, and this book provides a fantastic framework for improving clinicians' abilities to act intelligently in those situations. I recommend it to doctors, residents, nurses, and anyone who is involved in direct patient care. A must read.
~ Jeffrey S. Young

*****

Alexander L. Eastman, MD, MPH, FACS,
Lieutenant, Dallas Police Department (SWAT),
Interim Medical Director, The Trauma Center at Parkland
(UT Southwestern Medical Center)

In my experiences on SWAT, they don't pay us to get ready, but to always be ready. This book is an excellent resource to prepare the young surgeon to respond to inevitable intraoperative crises.

Ken Lipshy's *Crisis Management Leadership In The Operating Room* should help harden any operative team against compounding crisis through further error.*
~ Alexander L. Eastman

** Disclaimer: These statements represent the views of the endorser and do not necessarily express the views or policies of the Dallas Police Department.*

*****

Juan Sanchez, Cardiothoracic Surgeon, Director GME and Chair, Saint Agnes Hospital, Associate Professor of Surgery, Johns Hopkins Medicine, Baltimore, Maryland

This is truly a remarkable book for it delivers important concepts from a wide array of disciplines in a concise, readable format. It manages to put in perspective the real-world situations clinical practitioners actually face daily. Through realistic examples, this book explains why we behave the way we do in a crisis and how leaders can turn maladaptive behaviors to adaptive behaviors when it really counts. It lays out a framework useful for any safety-critical team to prepare for and prevent sudden adverse events and includes key references for the reader to pursue topics further.
~ Juan Sanchez

*****

Paul Lucha, MD, FAC, CAPT, MC, USN, Retired;
Department Head,
Department Surgery Navy Medical Center,
Portsmouth, VA

Dr. Lipshy has opened an important topic not only for surgery but medicine in general. An excellent review of the complexities surrounding crisis management. As a military surgeon, crisis frequently ensues surrounding combat trauma, specialty availability, and resource availability. Panic and errors can be avoided by recognizing and applying the concepts within this book. A must read for every surgeon and surgical leader.
~ Paul Lucha

*****

Douglas E. Paull, M.D.,
Director, Patient Safety Curriculum,
National Center for Patient Safety

Robin R. Hemphill, M.D., M.P.H.,
Chief Safety and Risk Awareness Officer Director,
National Center for Patient Safety

In his book *Crisis Management Leadership in the Operating Room – Prepare Your Team to Survive Any Crisis* Dr. Lipshy provides a pathway for teams to apply principles of crew resource management within high-reliability organizations to achieve exceptional leadership, communication, and teamwork during care of the surgical patient, especially during crises.

Dr. Lipshy provides the reader with a clear understanding of why unexpected crises may not be managed effectively due to lack of leadership, poor communication, and suboptimal teamwork using the established frameworks of high-reliability and crew resource management, punctuated by illustrative cases from aviation, other industries, healthcare, and the operating room.

Surgeons will enjoy and benefit from Dr. Lipshy's book as it takes them on a self-reflective journey on their own sometimes maladaptive behaviors or biases during unanticipated events, and includes effective techniques for overcoming these all too human tendencies. He reminds us that even the best physicians can have events conspire against them, and how they choose to react and interact can change everything. The importance of surgeon leadership in setting the tone in the operating room, developing a shared mental model, empowering other team members to voice concerns, and role modeling exemplary behavior under stress are highlighted and the reader is introduced to identifiable skills to enhance the quest to prevent, prepare for, and confront unanticipated crises in the operating room.

Crisis Management Leadership in the Operating Room – Prepare Your Team to Survive Any Crisis is a useful read for all operating room team members (surgeons, anesthesiologists, anesthesia providers, nurses, scrub techs, and others), patient safety officers, risk managers, and health care organizational leaders.
~ Douglas E. Paull and Robin R. Hemphill

*****

Robin L. Homolak, Nurse Manager, Operating Room,
Long Beach VA Healthcare System;
Advisor, ORNM Workgroup,
VA National Surgery Office

Surgeons rely on an Operating Room (O.R.) team that is experienced, competent, prepared, and focused with demonstrated expertise and knowledge of "Best Practices." The O.R. team expects the surgeon to be confident, technically skilled, professional, respectful, and in charge of the overall care of the patient. Together, this creates an "Environment of Safety"... and the patient deserves nothing less.

The role that we all play in the patient's care cannot be overlooked. Dr. Lipshy obviously has insight from both perspectives and the expertise to educate those of us who are passionate about our patients. My 34 years as an O.R. staff nurse and Manager in hospitals ranging from trauma centers to community hospitals have taught me the importance of a "tight knit team" not only for scheduled cases, but especially for crisis situations.

Having the courage to speak up with confidence is not part of every nurse's makeup, but when every individual on the team understands that his or her responsibility is to function optimally and professionally for every case, it takes the guesswork out of a crisis situation. The "predictability" factor for each person's role makes crisis management everyone's business.

A crisis is never routine, but when faced with the unexpected event in the O.R., if everyone's role becomes equally important and they work under the umbrella of respect, it gives the patient the best chance of a good outcome. Thank you, Dr. Lipshy, for helping all of us see the bigger picture. This book should be mandatory reading for surgeons as well as all other O.R. staff.
~ Robin L. Homolak

Foreword

Ajit K. Sachdeva, M.D., F.R.C.S.C., F.A.C.S.
Director, Division of Education
American College of Surgeons

The book, *Crisis Management Leadership in the Operating Room*, by Kenneth A. Lipshy, M.D., F.A.C.S., provides an excellent review of human cognitive errors, causes of errors, role of systems in preventing and mitigating errors, and education and training of surgical teams. National imperatives that necessitate focus on these domains are articulated well and examples from other high-reliability organizations are helpful in considering different strategies to improve safety in surgery. Topics of crisis management and effective leadership in the Operating Room environment are handled well. The key messages are succinctly articulated throughout the book.

This book should be a valuable resource to surgical leaders, practicing surgeons, surgery residents, and members of surgical teams. It should help in underscoring and extending further national efforts currently underway to deliver surgical care of the highest quality and promote safety. It should also be valuable to surgical educators as they design and introduce new training programs to address gaps in this field to harness the myriad opportunities ahead.

Disclaimer: The opinions expressed in this Foreword are those of the author and do not necessarily represent the official position of the American College of Surgeons.

Dedication

- To the patients who trust us to focus our undivided attention to their ailments, free from distraction and hesitation.

- To our surgical trainees who look to us as role models for their future success.

- To our surgical team cohorts who rely upon us to maintain unwavering composure during times of difficulty.

- To our families who trust us to support and love them wholeheartedly, free from distraction and hesitation.

- To our community who relies upon us to lead in a multitude of community organizations simultaneously while maintaining a busy clinical practice.

- To ourselves as surgical leaders to take upon ourselves these obligations yet maintain a stable mindset.

"The most concise but complete reference to the relationship of human error to the creation of and perpetuation of disasters… a well-constructed step-by-step approach how a surgical leader can teach and lead teams through crises, preventing them from becoming a disaster, using approaches manifested in our military and first responder forces."

~ Aubrey

Table of Contents

*****

Introduction

*****

PART ONE

Human Cognitive Error as a Pivotal Point in the Foundation of Operating Room Crises
75

*****

PART TWO

*****

PART THREE

Time Critical/Rapid Process Decision Making Events: Is Your Team Ready for its Next Crisis?

137

CONCLUSION

233

*****

Goal of this Book

After reading this book surgical leaders should be capable of teaching their O.R. team to:

1. Recognize how human error contributes to adverse events
2. Understand how system deficiencies can allow a simple error to progress to a catastrophe or how the system can be prepared to mitigate a mistake
3. Understand cognitive functions during normal and abnormal circumstances
4. Recognize that during a crisis the team will proceed through successful or self-destructive pathways determined by their ability to:
    - Control panic and dissociation
    - Establish clear lines of leadership and followership
    - Communicate effectively
    - Maintain situational awareness
    - Perform effective risk management strategies

Glossary

Adverse

Causing harm

Accident

An unforeseen and unplanned event or circumstance
An unfortunate event resulting especially from carelessness or ignorance

An unexpected happening causing loss or injury which is not due to any fault or misconduct on the part of the person injured but for which legal relief may be sought

Catastrophe

A momentous tragic event ranging from extreme misfortune to utter overthrow or ruin
Utter Failure

Crisis

An unstable or crucial time or state of affairs in which a

decisive change is impending; *especially* : one with the distinct possibility of a highly undesirable outcome
A situation that has reached a critical phase

Crisis Management

A (an organizational) crisis is a major, unpredictable event that threatens to harm an organization and its stakeholders. Although crisis events are unpredictable, they are not unexpected (Coombs, 1999). Crises can affect all segments of society—businesses, churches, educational institutions, families, non-profits and the government and are caused by a wide range of reasons. Although the definitions can vary greatly, three elements are common to most definitions of crisis:

1. A threat to the organization
2. The element of surprise
3. A short decision time (Seeger, Sellnow & Ulmer, 1998).

Disaster

A sudden calamitous event bringing great damage, loss, or destruction; a sudden or great misfortune or failure

Error

An act that through ignorance, deficiency, or accident departs from or fails to achieve what should be done

Used By permission. From *Merriam-Webster's Collegiate® Dictionary, 11th Edition* ©2013 by Merriam-Webster, Inc. (www.Merriam-Webster.com)

Preface

Ask yourself this question: "Have I prepared my O.R. team to handle any crisis they might encounter in the O.R., or are they destined to fail?"

As a leader in the operating room, your obligation is to assure that not only are ***your*** patients safe from expected undue harm, but also validate that your team is ready to handle any unexpected changes that may occur. Your obligation, to protect, centers not just on the patient but the team as well. You are expected to keep your team out of trouble. But, as Bear Grylls states, "If you fail to have a plan, you plan to fail." How can one possibly be ready for anything in the O.R. if one does not understand the implications of human cognitive error in the creation and perpetuation of a crisis or how the system can be effectively constructed to mitigate the full extent of the crisis or that failure to do so, inevitably leads the team to disaster?

Our responsibility as leaders begins well in advance of a crisis. We must be willing to assure that every member of the O.R. team is comfortable in their respective roles should a crisis occur and that can only occur by working with the team prior to the event. Once a crisis happens, it is too late.

Potentially lethal crises only happen a few times in one's career, so we will never experience enough of them to form habitual patterns of response. We must remember we cannot have a checklist for every scenario, but we can develop a plan to assure our team is mentally prepared to control panic, assess the situation at hand, determine the best course of action, *and act upon it*.

Once the crisis unfolds, our roles should be clear to us and our teammates. A local retired police officer once told me that the biggest mistake a police academy graduate can make is to believe that they are ready to move on to a different post-graduate role without using the tools taught to them. He warns graduates that they have to store everything in their *toolbox*. They have to remember that all the basic tools they learn are not simply there to get them to the next level, but to use frequently to adjust to changing scenarios and roles.

We need to learn the basics of proper response to unexpected threatening scenarios. Unfortunately it has been proven that experienced surgeons are overconfident in their ability to respond to an unexpected threatening situation. Unpublished data, regarding extreme environmental simulation with highly trained military professionals, reveals that providers acknowledged they were more confident than they should have been, and faced more anxiety than they originally anticipated they would have. It behooves us to give surgical teams tools for their toolbox to pull out when the unexpected event occurs. You simply cannot train or have a checklist for every specific scenario.

Retired Major General Robert F. Dees summarizes our roles and obligations as team leaders into several categories. Bob counsels and my commentary follows:

- "Positively affirm those in the midst of a crisis and give life to confused, scared, and disconsolate followers." We must be the stable factor in an unstable environment. It is our job to control chaos and panic.
- "Lead by example, taking action when paralysis and fear have immobilized others." You must train to avoid personal panic or paralysis in order to pull other team members from the grip of fear. If you are not able to do that, you must learn to step out of the way.
- "Mobilize external resources for the good of the cause, using their authority and influence to truly help their subordinates resolve the crisis." Inexperienced leaders frequently fail to ask for help early on, most likely due to their lack of appreciation for the magnitude or implications of the crisis.

- "Know when to stay out of the way, letting experts do their job in time sensitive settings of urgency." Often times it is better to let one's subordinates do what they are trained to do instead of delving into the details. Your job is to lead your team, activating the responses noted in the body of the text enclosed and come up with THE PLAN to save the mission, activate it and monitor the environment around you. If you are unable to do that because your role as surgeon is vital to save the patient's life, then call for backup to run the rest of the show. *Make that clear from the beginning.* As a surgeon, you cannot manage an exsanguinating hemorrhage and monitor a changing situation simultaneously.
- "Shield their subordinates from outside distractors, helping them focus on the crisis at hand." It is your prerogative to assure that those in the heat of a crisis are protected from outsiders during and after the event. Nothing demoralizes a team more than outsiders (or insiders) speaking negatively about the evolution of the event. [1]

In the heat of a disaster, Major General Bob Dees once told his subordinate "...it's not whether bad things happen that makes or breaks a commander. It's what he does with the hand he's dealt that really matters."[2]

So ask yourself the question: "Am I ready to lead my team given the hand we were dealt?"

O.R. Crisis Management Leadership Training courses should teach O.R. staff how simple, unexpected, cognitive errors or spontaneous events from "out-of-the-blue" can rapidly transform a normal situation into a crisis. When pre-existing conditions, imperfect system safety nets and further errors prevent mitigation at a salvageable state, a full-fledged disaster results.

An introduction to cognitive error and maladaptive responses to stress to the team should prepare them to engage in simulation training. By not providing this educational base, training will not show longevity simply because the trainees will not understand the origination of erroneous and maladaptive responses, and therefore remain unable to change the way they think and act during an intra-operative crisis.

No surgeon is born with the inherent knowledge to perform a complex surgical procedure. We learn the basics, then the steps in the procedure, one-by-one. The approach to Crisis Management Leadership should follow the same pattern.

This book is filled with advice from military, first responder, and wilderness survival experts which can easily be integrated into any simulation training to assure that staff understand why they have the option to perform as a combatant in any event, or that if they refuse that option, to allow the mission to fail.

Two recent surveys (one of American College of Surgeons members and another of American Society of Anesthesiologists members) have revealed the tragic consequences of errors and catastrophes on the physician psyche. While the patients are always at the heart of our patient safety concerns, as surgical leaders, we must be attuned to the second victim. Failure in the operating room, battlefield, airways, or any line of fire consistently results in negative team member psychological consequences. It is our responsibility to assure all teams are prepared for the unexpected.

The impact of a catastrophe: 2012 American Society of Anesthesiologists Survey

- 84% of Anesthesiologists were involved in at least one unanticipated death or serious injury of a perioperative patient over the course of his/her career.
- 70% experienced guilt, anxiety, and reliving of the event (88% requiring time to recover emotionally & 19% never fully recovered, 12% considered a career change)
- 67% believed that their ability to provide patient care was compromised in the first 4 hours subsequent to the event
- 7% were given time off.
- CONCLUSION: A perioperative catastrophe may have a profound and lasting emotional impact on the anesthesiologist involved and may affect his or her ability to provide patient care in the aftermath of such events.

Gazoni FM, Amato PE, Malik ZM, and Durieu ME. The impact of perioperative catastrophes on anesthesiologists: results of a national survey. *Anesth Analg*. 2012;114:(596-603) [3]

Introduction

Beep… beep… beep…

"What's going on up there? I am really trying to concentrate here and that racket is distracting us."

"Nothing, doc."

Beep… beep… beep… (muffled sounds above the anesthesia barrier)

"What is going on?"

"ETCO2 is up, but it's fine."

"If it's fine, can you keep it down!?"

"Hey, Nurse A., call Dr. Anesthesia."

"What is going on?"

"Nothing doc; I can't ventilate the patient well and need to bronch him!"

"Can you be a little quieter then?!"

"Mr. C… Dr. A. said he is in the endoscopy unit today and can't come down."

"Where is Dr. B? I need some help."

CRNA C walks in. "What's up? Oh, that ETCO2 monitor has been having problems. Didn't biomed fix it?"

"Hey! What is going on?!"

"Nothing, Doc. What's the abdomen pressure?"

"I don't know! Nurse, why can't I see that monitor? What's the pressure?"

"The intra-abomen pressure monitor hasn't been working right. Let me try another cable and different tubing."

"Are you kidding me?! What's the ETCO2?"

"It's 80."

"What?! This isn't a time to be messing around guys. What do we need to do?"

"Nothing; it's probably the monitor."

"Doctor, the abdomen pressure is 12."

"What is happening now?"

"Scoping the patient and getting some nasty stuff out and ETCO2 is 100."

"Great! Nurse, can you pull up the pre-op chest xray?"

"The x-ray report says, 'Right lower lobe infiltrate, cannot rule out atelectasis or pneumonia."

"What? Hey, Mr. B, why did I not know that?"

"Well, sir, I sent you a text yesterday evening around 6 p.m."

"Great. Did you guys get a blood gas yet?"

"Working on it right now, Doc; waiting for some blood gas tubes."

"Well, do I need to quit now before I go across the IMA?"

"No, everything is Fi…n……XXXX! What just happened?!"

"What is going on now?!"

"Nurse, *get Dr. A here now!*"
BEEP… BEEP… BEEP… BEEP… BEEP….

"What is going on?!"

"PO2 is down, ETCO2 is 150 and the pressure is reading 60 systolic!"

"What?! I can see an aortic pulse! Looks fast!"

"XXXX… Can't tell if he has a CO2 embolus, PE, Pneum……., I don't know…..are you loosing blood, Doc?"

"I thought you said the ETCO2 monitor was broken?"

Dr. A walks in. "What the… No, the monitor's fine, they came and fixed it yesterday… That is probably right. You need to stop this operation now!"

"'Can't! 'got some bleeding here. Where's that coming from? 'Can't stop. You are going to need to give some blood. We need to open… I can't see!"

"Nurse! What is going on?! I said I can't see!!!"

Nurse: " The CO2 tank is empty and we are having problems changing it out."

"What? Did we get a type and screen? Did you order anything?"

"Guys, I don't know, that's your job, I can't do everything, I have to stop this… that's a lot of blood! What's the BP?"

"Hey! What's the BP? Is there anyone up there?"

"Doctor, Can you see we are have a problem here? You need to leave us alone."
Beep… Beep… Beep…

"Someone, get some help in here. Stop leaving the room! I am trying to open here! Hey you, what are you doing standing there? Help us! I can't see a thing. Why aren't you helping me? Suction's not working."

"You've filled all our canisters, Doc!"

Beep… Beep… Beep… ______________________________

"What happened to the lights?!"

"Truck backed into the transformer, emergency power should be on in second."

"I can't see!"

"Oh my, this is bad, really bad! … *This man is going to die!* I don't know what to do, what to do, get me some help! *Why are you just standing there? Help me!* This man's going to die if you guys don't do something fast!"…

Evolution of an Error, to an Adverse Event, to a Crisis, to Survival, or a Disaster

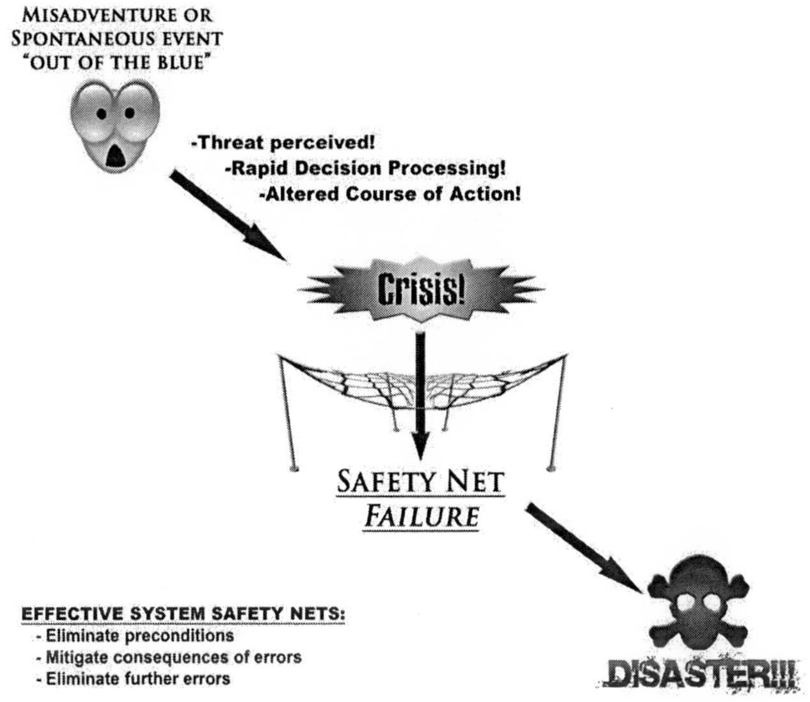

Figure 1 Evolution of a Crisis in the O.R. In this book, the reader shall learn how simple unexpected cognitive errors or spontaneous events from "out-of-the-blue" can rapidly transform a crisis situation into a disaster when pre-existing conditions, imperfect system safety nets, and further errors prevent mitigation at a salvageable state. The time to learn these lessons is *before* they happen.

On any given day, a seemingly minor error or spontaneous event, *out-of-the-blue,* coupled with underlying systemic issues, subsequent mistakes, and faulty system safety-nets, will evolve into an intra-operative O.R. Crisis (IORC) with the potential to mushroom into a full-blown disaster (Figure 1).

What was that error? It could be any of thousands that happen every day: wrong device, wrong patient, wrong side, wrong sponge count, failed equipment, missing device, transected organ or vessel, wrong medication, missing progressive downward trend, esophageal intubation, etc.

What is a crisis? A personal determination of what constitutes a crisis without a specific definition can create confusion. Without a specific designation of what situation can be designated a crisis, the interpretation of any event by those involved fully depends on their perception of the event and their prior experience in coping with that type of situation. One person's crisis may just be an average day in another person's life. For an average person, in an average community, walking outside to find projectiles flying at them would constitute a crisis, but this may be an average day in the life of someone in the military or police force. For an M.D. walking into a room with blood transfusion bags hanging by the dozen, alarms blasting and multiple conversations occurring simultaneously, that may be a shock or just an average day.

An **adverse event** is an occurrence that causes harm to something. In of itself, just because something has an adverse consequence, does not by definition make it a crisis.

In 1963 Hermann devised a model to conceptualize the origination of organizational crises. While many such models for organizational disasters are available, similar models for other circumstances are not readily available, but clearly one can apply these same principles in most crisis situations.

As seen in Figure 2, below, in most situations, for an event to evolve into a **crisis**, four elements are usually required:

1. Surprise! This was not expected. You were caught off guard. The team is suddenly confronted by an unanticipated and unfamiliar circumstance. Most likely they were functioning in a routine with expectations that things will proceed as usual. This new event is now something unfamiliar and outside the team's predictable pattern. On a side note, experts mentally anticipate the unexpected, so when the unexpected occurs they are mentally prepared for it and can analyze the situation in a non-stressed environment. That is how military and police "soldiers" survive in an uncertain world.
2. Threat to the organization, team, or mission. A surgical team's mission is to help patients assume an improved productive life as quickly as possible, and

to assure we have created no harm. During a crisis this high priority goal is clearly jeopardized. It is clear to the team that this threat is a discrepancy between the desired and existing states. The severity of the threat is related to the probability of loss to the mission.

3. Time-critical, rapid processing decision times Crisis, in of its nature, requires that processes occur rapidly to avoid harm. It is this same rush to complete the task that can create a paradoxical sluggishness in an individual or group. This time pressure can either create decisional paralysis or responses that occur too rapidly to gather adequate and appropriate information and then analyze it. This time compression is what makes responses to crises susceptible to cognitive error as will be seen later.
4. Transformation is needed. We need to make a change in our current process, procedure, course of actions, etc.. If we don't change anything during the course of events, then we end up with a failure. Typically there is an overload of the baseline state. Those immediately involved in the situation find themselves with too many unknown variables (not enough accurate information), information overload, too many tasks, not enough staff, not enough working equipment and so on, to manage the situation successfully without some changes. [4-6]

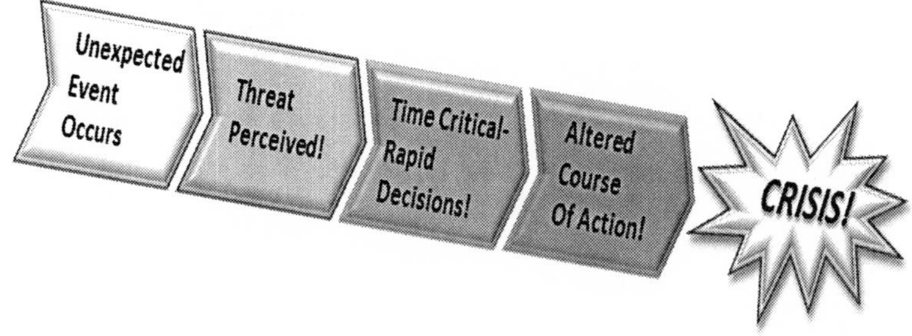

Figure 2 Evolution of a Crisis

An unexpected error, accident, or other surprise occurs followed by crisis evolution including a threat, rapid processing time requirements, and finally the need to alter the current course. Depending on preexisting conditions, team and system safety net responses (such as crisis training), the outcome will either be survival or a disaster.

Adapted from:

Seeger, M. W.; Sellnow, T. L., & Ulmer, R. R. Communication, organization and crisis". *Communication Yearbook*. 1998;21: 231-275 [4]

Venette, S. J. *Risk Communication in a High Reliability Organization: APHIS PPQ's Inclusion of Risk in Decision Making*. Ann Arbor, MI: UMI Proquest Information and Learning; 2003. [5]

Disasters, Catastrophes

These terms broadly describe sudden events causing great damage, loss, destruction, misfortune, or significant failure. In an organizational sense a disaster happens on a larger scale and has a widespread impact, while a crisis tends to be a more local event with less overall impact. The goal in the end is to survive and remain functional. One of the better definitions for measuring the impact of a crisis or disaster is by the U.S. Coast Guard (USCG) in its handbook on risk management. The USCG classifies levels of severity of events, in terms of degree of impact on the system, worst to least severe, as:

1. Catastrophic—Complete mission failure, death, or loss of system.
2. Major—Major mission degradation, severe injury, minor occupational illness, or major system damage.
3. Significant—Minor mission degradation, injury, minor occupational illness, or minor system damage.
4. Minimal—Less than minor mission degradation, injury, occupational illness, or minor system damage.
5. None—No impact to personnel or mission outcome.

COMMANDANT INSTRUCTION 3500.3

How Did We Not See That Coming?

Crises in the operating room have a potential for horrendous consequences for the patient and the team if the team response is not successful. Not all disasters are unexpected. Sometimes a team is hopeful but a case may not result in patient survival. This may occur when a patient is moribund, the team and patient fully understand that the patient may not survive, but the surgeon feels he can save the patient and the patient wishes to proceed anyway.

When the patient dies on the Operating Room table, it is a catastrophic event emotionally for the team. It was not that unexpected, though. On that note, not all that is unexpected is a crisis. When a surgeon unexpectedly finds a simple adhesive band as a cause of obstruction at exploration, greatly limiting the expected operative time in a relaparotomy, that is fortuitous.

Crises by nature are unexpected and typically they are unexpected because:

1. Something that was supposed to happen didn't.
2. Something that was not supposed to happen did.
3. Something simply flies in out-of-the-blue that no one could have predicted.

As seen in Figure 3, crises in the operating room can arise internally to the O.R. or institution (i.e. retained sponge, wrong or expired implant, arrest or exsanguination) or externally (earthquake, tornado, flood, act of war). The ones an O.R. team typically encounters, and the ones to be described here, are internal crises—those that arise from human error, system error, or inherent patient factors (the response overall, though, would not be that different if the threat was external).

The most common origins of an O.R. crisis include:

1. Unrecognized incremental evolution of smaller adverse events.
2. Missing the warning signs of an impending problem.

3. Unexpected, sudden change in patient condition due to something someone on the team did, an inherent patient problem, or equipment/product problem or reaction. [7]

Even in external disasters, post-recovery analysis frequently reveals gaps in the system preparation; hence in reality there was an internal factor that went unnoticed. Even if external, the response to a crisis should be basically the same.

Now that the crisis has occurred, how do we (the team and patient) survive? How do we prevent the crisis from becoming a disaster? Rely on our instincts? Pull out the crisis check sheets? Call in the "old dog?"

Internal vs. External Source of Crises

1. Internal
    a. Equipment malfunction
    b. Team-retained sponge, implant error
    c. Patient—Malignant Hyperthermia, Arrest, Hemorrhage
2. External
    a. Earthquake
    b. Tornado
    c. Flood
    d. Act of Violence/War

Common Origins of O.R. Crises

1. Incremental evolution of smaller adverse events
2. Missing the warning signs of an impending problem
3. Unexpected sudden change in patient condition due to something someone on the team did or inherent patient problem, or equipment/product problem or reaction.

Crises Are Unexpected Because:

1. Something that was supposed to happen didn't.
2. Something that was not supposed to happen did.

Figure 3 "Sources of Crises and Why They are Unexpected"
Adapted in part with permission from:
Gaba DM, Fish KJ, Howard SK. *Crisis Management in Anesthesiology*. New York, NY: Churchill Livingstone; 1994.[7]

Scope of the Problem: Just How Bad Could It Be? What Is the Incidence of Errors in Medicine?

On April 22, 1982, ABC 20/20 aired a program titled *The Deep Sleep: 6,000 will die or suffer brain damage* stipulating that every year 6,000 Americans die or suffer brain damage relating to anesthesia accidents. Immediately afterwards, in 1983, the British Royalty Society of Medicine and the Harvard School of Medicine jointly sponsored a symposium on anesthesia deaths. Soon thereafter, in 1984, the International Symposium on Preventable Anesthesia Mortality and Morbidity was held in Boston, which was soon followed by the American Society of Anesthesiologists establishment of the Anesthesia Patient Safety Foundation. [8] Unfortunately, little further attention was paid to the issue of adverse events in patient care for another seventeen years.

The 1999 Institute of Medicine report, "To Err is Human" (and 2001 sequel, "Crossing the Quality Chasm"), citing "at least 44,000 Americans die each year as a result of medical errors," and "the total national costs… of preventable adverse events... are estimated to be between $17 billion and $29 Billion," stimulated an ongoing debate on how to create a safer health care environment in our country [9-10]

Simultaneously, in 1999, Gawande wrote, "To much of the public, and certainly to the lawyers and media, medical error is fundamentally a problem of bad doctors ... Mistakes do happen. We tend to think of them as aberrant. They are, however, anything but." [11-12] The Joint commission followed these reports, two years later, with the Universal Protocol guidelines for preventing wrong site, wrong procedure protocol, providing guidance for the healthcare industry to potentially prevent these devastating occurrences. [13] Surprisingly, many are not aware either of the multiple reports of preventable error statistics that had been published years prior to the Institute of Medicine studies, or that the data presented in the Institute of Medicine report most likely underestimates the true frequency of such errors due to its retrospective nature. [14-17]

While health care facilities overall are extremely complicated, operating rooms are considerably more complex due to the large number of groups that must be coordinated to assure that safe, efficient, affordable health care is administered, thus creating an environment that is even more prone than others to adverse events that could potentially progress to a crisis and typically have more catastrophic results than those that occur elsewhere in the healthcare facility. [16-18] A recent two-decade review of paid malpractice claims and judgments uncovered 9,744 claims from 1990-2010 for a total of $1.3 billion paid. These injuries included mortalities (6.6%), permanent injuries (32.9%), temporary injury (59.2%), retained foreign body (49.8%), wrong procedure (25.1%), wrong site (24.8%) and wrong patient in (0.3%). In the authors' estimate, given that 70% of patients do not file a claim, patients potentially suffer 4,082 surgical adverse events a year in the United States. [19]

A single study on Ophthalmology Procedures, in New York between 2001 and 2005, noted there were 62 incidents of wrong surgery among 900,000 eye procedures (or 69 per million or 10 times the quality-defect standard of Six Sigma accepted by manufacturing industry). [20] Similar to the medical field, Aviation Safety crash analyses reveal that human error accounts for over 80% of adverse incidents related to aircraft crashes. This fact bears true in almost any safety inspection following an incident, accident, disaster, etc. in any field. Simply put, most crises and subsequent disasters in high pressure organizations are preceded in the majority of cases by an act of human error. [21-27]

<u>$1.3 billion paid in 9,744 malpractice claims reviewed from 1990-2010</u>

6.6% mortalities, 32.9% permanent injuries,

59.2% temporary injury,

49.8% retained foreign body, 25.1% wrong procedure,

24.8%wrong site,

and 0.3% wrong patient

Current Status of Operating Rooms during a Crisis: "Just how safe is this plane?"

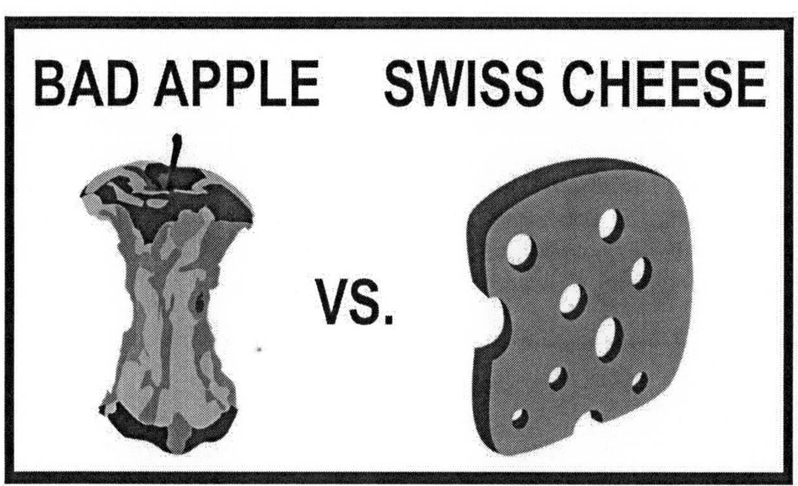

Figure 4 Bad Apple vs. Swiss Cheese: whose fault is it when things go wrong in the Operating Room? The surgeons, Surgical Team, or Hospital System?

> *"How efficient a life saving station have you in your operating room?*
> *Is it safe for me to collapse or have respiratory or cardiac arrest while undergoing an abdominal operation under your care?"*
>
> Dr. Wayne Babcock, June, 1924, at the Third Annual Congress of Anesthetists, the American, Mid-Western and Chicago Anesthetists in Joint Meeting with the National Anesthesia Research Society, Auditorium Hotel, Chicago [29-30]

For decades before and after the Institute of Medicine reports, volumes of literature have been compiled regarding the origin of an individual's mental mistakes in industry, as well as how systems' roles and responsibilities in complex industries could potentially prevent propagation of that mistake into a disaster. From these reports, two camps, on who is responsible for crisis evolution, have evolved:

1. The "Bad-Apple" proponents
2. The System Design proponents. [28]

Consequently, there have also been multiple reports in several fields on how the response of an individual or of a group to a disaster can either dampen or accelerate the effects of the crisis. This exact question was brought up by Dr. Wayne Babcock in June 1924, at the Third Annual Congress of Anesthetists, the American, Mid-Western and

Chicago Anesthetists in Joint Meeting with the National Anesthesia Research Society, Auditorium Hotel, Chicago, *"How efficient a life saving station have you in your operating room? Is it safe for me to collapse or have respiratory or cardiac arrest while undergoing an abdominal operation under your care?"* [29-30]

Nine decades later, the answer remains obscure. Minimal education exists in a concise format towards orientation of surgical teams regarding the relationship of:

1. Human errors to instigation of IORC
2. System design in mitigation of errors
3. Exacerbation or mitigation of the overall effects of an IORC based on the team's response.

In a 2009 survey of Australian surgeons, the surgeons acknowledged that, while in most situations surgeons are confident and able to make rational, quick decisions, when the unexpected crisis happens, their character "crumbles" and they are unable to handle the stress. The surgeons noted that while most high-risk industries introduce stress and crisis management training to their staff to prepare them to handle untoward events, the surgical field in general does not prepare surgeons for dealing with a stressful crisis. [31]

Since the 1980's, the aviation industry has conducted a significant amount of training for their crews to assure they are ready for most crisis situations. [21, 24, 25, 27] Additionally, over the past several decades, our anesthesia cohorts have progressively integrated programs designed to improve performance during an anesthesia crisis. [7, 18, 32-34]

There is scant literature on the incidence of crisis scenario occurrences in operating rooms, but in a 2005 review of 163,403 Thai Anesthesia cases, there were 212 cardiac arrests (30.8/10,000), 171 deaths (28.3/10,000), 44 esophageal intubations (4.1/10,000), 521 desaturation events (31.9/10,000), 243 difficult intubations (22.5/10,000), 34 failed intubations (3.1/10,000), 17 anaphylactic reactions (2.1/10,000), but zero malignant hyperthermia cases. In the multicenter study of general anesthesia of 1990, of 17,201 operations, there was a 5% incidence of severe events. In a study by Cooper, there was an incidence of 3% of serious events. [35-37]

The rarity of these events and lack of consistent formal crisis management training may explain why anesthesia studies have shown that a) experience does not prevent failure, and b) senior providers make mistakes during IORC. This should be alarming considering that in these same studies a) in 50% of IORC, the signs were non-specific, resulting in a delay in the determination of the cause and appropriate corrective action, and b) during complex life threatening crises, the team is forced to rely upon cognitive tasking far beyond the information processing capacity of the human brain. Given the rarity of these events surgeons and surgical teams should be prepared to handle these in a similar manner as the aviation industry. [32-34, 38-41]

Why should we worry? Here's why:

1. These events are rare!
2. Experience does not prevent failure—senior providers make mistakes during IORC!
3. Signs are frequently non-specific, resulting in a delay in the determination of the cause and appropriate corrective action, creating more team stress.
4. The team is usually forced to rely upon cognitive tasking far beyond the information processing capacity of the human brain.
5. Only 10-20% of people have an ability to remain calm in a crisis situation!

In most fields, human cognitive error research has provided staff education with subsequent error, crisis, and disaster reduction. Given that medical errors have not been eliminated and that newer trainees reportedly are not trained as effectively to handle crises, surgical teams need to increase their understanding of human factors in the creation of surgical-medical errors, fortify the system design to prevent propagation of errors to a crisis or disaster, and train to calmly handle a crisis using realistic simulation scenarios.

This training is needed desperately. Not planning for the worst case scenario, regardless how infrequently it will be encountered, is planning for failure during a crisis. The question remains how to motivate the field to push forward.

Scope of the Problem: Surgeon Preparation; "Looks like a storm's a- brewin!" "Are the captain and crew ready?" "Hey! Who's flying this plane?"

While there has been continued progress in the direction of assessment of communication, professionalism, and surgical skills of surgical providers in more structured formats and even progressive discussion regarding the psychological after-effects of OR errors and crises, there has been little team training in OR crisis intervention. [42-43] To make matters worse, in a 2010 report by Chung et al, it was noted that 25% of the residents' operative experience consisted of closed procedures and trauma operative experience decreased by 50%. Their conclusion was that *"Lack of operative trauma hurts intra-operative crisis management and decision making. "* [44]

Several other reports have also noted that the changes in the construct of Surgery Residency programs have reduced both total number of operative cases as well as the complexity of the cases performed. [45-48] This information is even more alarming when one takes into account the 2009 National survey of residents by Yeo, et al, revealing that 27.5% of residents did not feel comfortable performing operations independently and 63.8% felt they needed to complete fellowship training. [49] One hundred twenty-five PGY5 surgery resident responders to Pugh's 2010 survey revealed that residents did not feel they were adequately prepared for instrument or suture use/selection. Given that these are needs so easily conveyed in textbooks and in the operating room theater, one could infer that crisis management training is even less engrained. [50]

IORC have the potential for disastrous consequences if the team possesses poor coping mechanisms. Effective system design coupled with preemptive team training should prevent propagation of an IORC to a disaster (the point where significant damage has occurred).

Given that medical errors may not be decreasing in frequency and that newer trainees are reportedly not trained as effectively to handle crises, the surgical community has a need to increase its understanding of human factors in the creation of surgical-medical errors, fortify the system design to prevent propagation of that error to a crisis situation, and train surgical teams to calmly handle a crisis using realistic simulation scenarios.

This training is needed desperately.
Not planning for the worst case scenario, regardless how infrequently it will be encountered, is planning for failure during a crisis.
The question remains how to motivate the field to push forward.

The Sections that Follow Should Prepare Surgical Teams to:

1. Comprehend the influence of human cognitive errors on the instigation of O.R. crises—the various reasons people seem to do stupid things—
2. Understand systems' role in mitigation of errors—how an organization can prepare itself to minimize the damage to the patient, team and organization—
3. Learn beneficial vs. detrimental surgical team responses to an operating room crisis thereby training for mental preparedness to function in a systematic, panic controlled fashion and avoid a disaster

"Managing Risk should be a continuous and developing process that pervades our strategy. It must be integrated into our culture, our approach to problem solving and our decision making."
Admiral Michael G Mulen www.safetycenter.navy.mil.com

"Our sailors volunteered to join the Navy and our program because they sought to associate themselves with an elite community, doing challenging work, for noble causes. They don't want to be associated with an organization that lacks integrity, and they really don't want poor performance rationalized with lame excuses."
Admiral Kirkland H Donald, Director Naval Nuclear Propulsion,
Deputy Administrator,
National Nuclear Security Administration, June 2008

"Learn from the mistakes of others—
you can never live long enough
to make them all yourself."
~ *Unknown*

"Always expect something to go wrong.
Believe me, if you're wrong, you're not disappointed.
If you're right, you're ready for it."

Flanagan J. *Ranger's Apprentice: Book 7: Erak's Ransom.* New York, NY. Philomel Books (Penguin); 2007: 220.

PART ONE

Human Cognitive Error as a Pivotal Point in the Foundation of Operating Room Crises

The Many Ways the Human Brain Can Screw Things Up

In virtually all complex industries, the majority of adverse events are initiated or propagated by a wide variety of *human errors*.

> **er ror:** an act that through ignorance, deficiency, or accident departs from or fails to achieve what should be done
> http://www.merriam-webster.com/

Human error has been implicated in the creation of adverse events in the majority of most complex industries.

In aviation, multiple sources in the pre-Crew Resource (Cockpit) Management (CRM) era report human error as a cause of aviation incidents in over 50-80% of cases. [24-27]

The Institute of Medicine and other reports from 2000 estimated that medical errors resulted in 44,000 to 98,000 preventable deaths and 1,000,000 excess injuries each year in U.S. hospitals alone. [9, 51] A 2001 study of VA medical centers estimated that for roughly every 10,000 patients admitted to the subject hospitals, one patient died who would have lived for three months or more in good cognitive health had "optimal" care been provided. [14, 52]

Whether human error is the cause of adversity or if human error is the result of systems issues will be discussed later. Having said that, as will be outlined in the chapter on systems roles in the mitigation of human error, human error is a major component in the majority of organizational adverse events and crises. To move forward into the role systems have in preventing crises without fully understanding the origin of human error, would be somewhat premature.

Was that error a Slip, a Mistake, or a Violation?

Why Bad Things Happen: Human Error Theory
What Is Human Error?

Reason defines human error as "failure of planned actions to achieve their desired goals—without the intervention of some unforeseeable event." Failure occurs when the following events occur:

A. Slips, lapses, trips, or fumbles: the plan was adequate but actions failed to produce the desired goal due to unintended failures of execution, attention, or perception.
B. Mistakes: mental process involved in assessing the available information, the planning, formulating of intentions and judging the likely consequences of the planned actions by either misapplication or complete violation of known good rules, or the application of bad rules.
C. Violations: deviations from standard operating procedures either deliberately or erroneously. Deliberate acts are either ***malevolent*** or ***non-malevolent***. Routine violations usually involve corner-cutting, short-cuts that can become habitual. This usually happens when standard operating procedures seem to take longer than necessary. Many "violations" are deemed to be "necessary" in order to get the job done, such as when inadequate tools or training exist. Optimizing violations happen for the thrill, such as driving too fast. [53]

In the late 1990s, the US Navy developed a process to investigate maintenance error on naval aircraft, called Human Factors Analysis and Classification System—Maintenance Extension (HFACS-ME). They classified violations at three levels:

1. Routine – A maintainer engages in practices condoned by management that bend the rules.
2. Situational – A maintainer strays from accepted procedures to save time, bending a rule.
3. Exceptional – A maintainer willfully breaks standing rules, disregarding the consequences.

A United Kingdom Flight Safety Committee report in 2004 determined the top ten causes of the maintenance mishaps. Three of the top ten are clear cut violations. These ten violations may not come as a surprise to investigators of adverse events in any profession as the scenarios are familiar in just about any environment.

1. Failure to follow published technical data or local instructions
2. Using unauthorized procedure not referenced in technical data
3. Failure to document maintenance properly in maintenance records, work package
4. Performing an unauthorized modification to the aircraft

5. Supervisors accepting non-use of technical data or failure to follow maintenance instructions
6. Inattention to detail/complacency
7. Incorrectly installed hardware on an aircraft/engine
8. Failure to conduct a tool inventory after completion of the task
9. Personnel not trained or certified to perform the task
10. Ground support equipment improperly positioned for the task [53, 26]

Why Does Human Error Exist in Any Organization?

As noted above, two theories on the development of crises and industrial disasters prevail:

1. Bad Apple: when a mistake or error occurs resulting in a disaster, that responsible person is a "bad-apple." Human error causes bad accidents; failures are unpleasant, unsuspected surprises and complex systems are basically safe.
2. Systems Theory: Any adverse outcomes of individual acts are a result of a faulty system. [28]

Most clinicians are unaware of the reports from the 1970s trying to explain the existence of human errors in medical care as a primary cause of adverse events. In a Hastings Center Report from 1975, Gorovitz and MacIntyre stated that errors arise from ignorance or the "willfulness of negligence" i.e., ineptitude. [38, 54] Atul Gawande (World Health Organization Director of the "Safe Surgery Saves Lives" Initiative in 2006), described this mentality when he stated that "fallibility comes from both failures of ignorance and failures of ineptitude, the latter being failure to deliver on existing knowledge. Both can occur in surgery, but 'ineptitude' plays a substantial part." [55]

In a discussion regarding the nuclear power industry, Lee simply stated that "people don't always do what they are supposed to do. Some employees have negative attitudes to safety which adversely affect their behavior. This undermines the system of multiple defenses that an organization constructs." [22] If these theories are true, then all errors in industry are theoretically the result of planned out actions and are not due to any inherent human cognitive dysfunction. The assumption with the "bad-apple" theory is that complex systems are essentially safe and a single individual can create havoc on their own, resulting in a bad outcome. With these premises, it is more convenient to condemn individuals or the team for a complication, than it is to attempt to understand the underlying issues responsible for a poor outcome.

As noted by Vincent, "once outcomes have been correctly adjusted for patient risk factors, the remaining variance is *assumed to be explained by the individual surgical skill.* This view neglects a wide range of factors that have been found to be of importance in achieving safe high quality performance in other high risk environments." [56]

EFFECTS OF HINDSIGHT BIAS

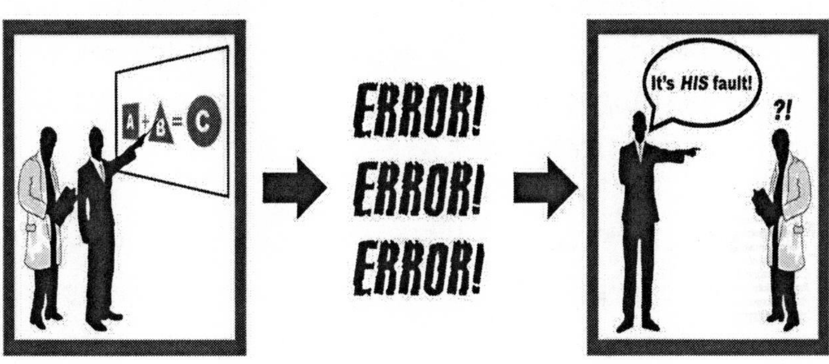

Figure 5 Effects of Hindsight Bias after accident occurrence. Regardless of all the planning prior to any event, a reactive investigational review assumes the individual is totally responsible for the negative outcome. It is easier to condemn individuals or a team than to understand the underlying issues responsible for a bad outcome. Assuming error can be "explained by the individual Surgical Skill" neglects a wide range of factors "that have been found to be of importance in achieving safe high-quality performance in other high risk environments."

Adapted from Vincent C, Moorthy K, Sarker SK, Chang A, Darzi AW. Systems approach to surgical quality and safety. *Ann Surg.* 2004;239(4):475-482. [29]

This mindset is extremely common in medical error assessment. Shortly after the introduction of the laparoscopic cholecystectomy in the 1990s, it was recognized that laparoscopic common bile duct injuries (LCBDI) occurred at twice the rate seen previously during the open cholecystectomy procedures (LCBDI rate between 0.4 - 0.7%). The early assumption was that when an LCBDI injury occurred, it should be considered practice below the standard of care, and that experienced surgeons did not have these complications. [57]

In 2003, Dr. Way and Hunter's group reviewed 252 LCBDI videos. Instead of finding that the surgeons were operating under poor conditions, they realized that in 97% of cases of LCBDI, the surgeon simply did not recognize the injury. In only 3% of cases there were faults in technical skill. They performed one of the first human factor approaches to this issues and their experts concluded that, in the majority of cases, there was a visual perception illusion. [58]

The conclusion of their video review study was that errors associated with LCBDI were typically due to the surgeon not perceiving the error was about to occur. The surgeon seemed to be subconsciously committed to an assumption that everything was normal in spite of the obvious fact, retrospectively, all was not normal. The surgeons appeared to be totally unaware of the events as they were unfolding in front of them. It was as if they were completely blinded to the situation. Corrective feedback after identification of an ***irregularity*** should have occurred, but it did not.

For one to understand the needs for dealing with this stress, one first needs to fully comprehend the human cognitive factors responsible for error creation. [59] Given the danger in any deviation in a laparoscopic procedure, and the known inherent pitfalls of laparoscopy, it is easy to see there is simply no threshold for allowing the addition of human cognitive error to creep undetected into these cases.

> Faults with laparoscopy such as loss of haptic perception, loss of stereoscopy, and limitations of perspective laparoscopy require greater concentration and place greater mental stress on surgeons than open surgery. These inherent issues, compounded with poor coping strategies, highlight the need for effective training in intraoperative stress-coping strategies. [59]

The first question most ask when reading this is, "How is that possible? How could any experienced surgeon simply not see something that is right there?" To answer that question, one simply has to recall the classic 1999 Harvard experiment by Simons and Chabris, where observers are asked to count how many times a basketball is being passed around. At the end of the experiment, 50% of observers totally miss that a "Gorilla" passes through the room and stands in the middle of the players for several seconds before moving off to the side. It was as if the Gorilla was totally invisible. According to Simons and Chabris, "We are missing a lot of what goes on around us. We have no idea we are missing so much." [61]

In his book, *Thinking, Fast and Slow* Daniel Kahneman summarized this: "The gorilla study illustrates two important facts about our minds: we can be blind to the obvious and we are also blind to our blindness." [62]

Daniel Kahneman defined heuristics as "a simple procedure that helps find adequate, though often imperfect, answers to difficult questions." [62] As will be shown later, humans' innate habit of missing the "gorilla" in the room can be costly in terms of dollars and lives lost.

Errors of cognition that can result in human error fall in to one of the following categories that will be explained in detail below.

1. Heuristics (illusions, ambiguity)
2. Confirmation Bias / Fixation
3. Causation / Over-steering (the hands follow the eyes)
4. Complacency—Risk Taking
5. Environmental Awareness—Common Sense
6. Distractions / Environmental Stressors

Heuristic Influence on Cognition: "Hey, where did that triangle come from?"

Simply stated, prior to making a conscious decision, your mind takes in visual, auditory, and haptic perceptive clues from the environment (input). These clues, plus your subconscious long-term memory of similar experiences, are then processed into a conscious outcome (output).

Rasmussen distinguished human performance at three levels (See Figure 6):

1. Skill-based (SB)
2. Rule-based (RB)
3. Knowledge-based (KB)

When looking at the transition from automatic subconscious functions to deliberate conscious actions, the human mind transitions between the three levels of thinking. We use the *skill-based* processes much of the time at the automatic subconscious level. These are the routine actions carried out mostly without much thought (the things we do on a routine basis such as driving to work or home).

At some point we have to move to an intermediate *rule-based* level. Usually there is a recognized change in the situation. Hopefully it is a problem we have dealt with previously and have training to deal with it. We apply memorized rules to automatically deal with the situation.

There is a transition back and forth between conscious and subconscious processing. If all else fails and we get to the point where we recognize we have not solved the problem we are forced to move to the conscious effort known as *knowledge-based* problem solving. We acknowledge that all the automatic rules we applied did not work and now we have to consider the issue at hand more thoroughly and come up with a solution. This is a slower process that works fine if we have time and luxury of trial and error, but in an emergency this can be an issue. In a crisis we have inaccurate, incomplete information, and unfortunately the conscious mind can only handle small bits of information simultaneously. *It is said we cannot handle more than two to three distinct items at a time.* Our attention drops issues as we move back and forth from one problem to another.

"It is said that we cannot handle more than two to three distinct items at one time."

Considering this, it is understandable how confusing things appear when we toss in fear, shock, and denial. Trying to come up with novel solutions is virtually impossible in this scenario, but unfortunately, subconscious rule-based efforts no longer work at this point.

The best example is driving to work. Most of this process is at the subconscious skill-based level (awareness of traffic patterns, the usual route, acceleration and deceleration). As we move between the conscious and subconscious notations of traffic we use rule based behavior (someone is driving too slow and we need to get around or someone is coming up fast behind us and we need to get over). If some change occurs unexpectedly we have to shift rapidly through rule based and knowledge based efforts to assess and resolve the problem. If it is as simple as a sign noting a road closure or traffic ahead, we have time to work through our options. If suddenly there is a large animal in the road and the truck in front of us slams on his brakes and is in the middle of the road and there are large trucks on the side and behind us, we have to use thoughts and actions we may not be prepared for and have no time for trial and error. [53, 63]

Mental processing, with its potential pitfalls, is not easy in unexpected situations. Mental distortions, to be described soon, are augmented when this processing has to be done rapidly under pressure. The techniques for managing volumes of information and developing appropriate plans of action will be discussed later.

SKILL-BASED PERFORMANCE
(sub-conscious)

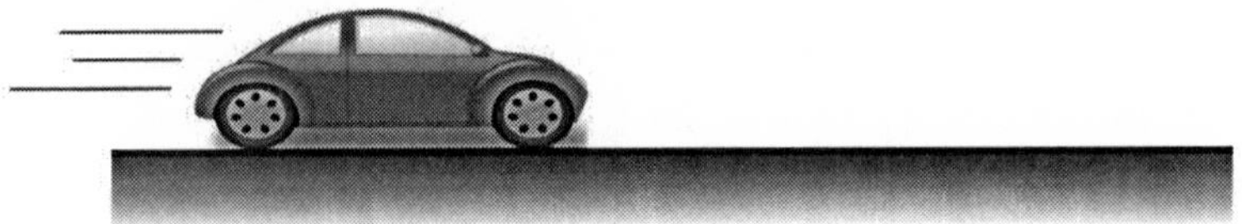

RULE-BASED PERFORMANCE
(semi-conscious)

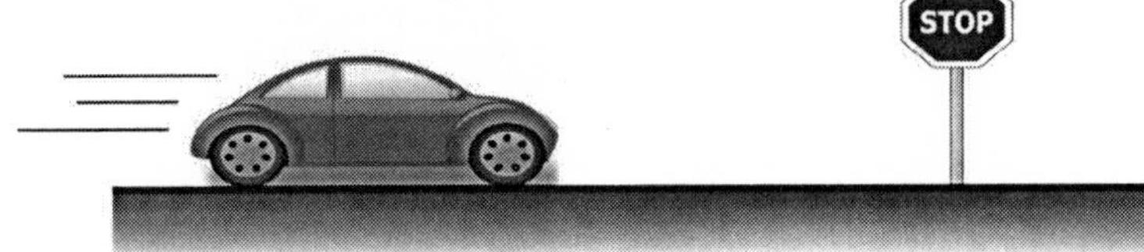

KNOWLEDGE-BASED PERFORMANCE
(conscious)

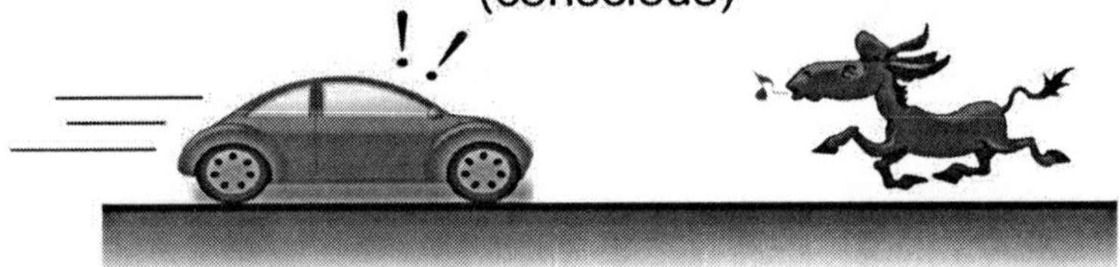

Figure 6 Levels of Performance based on level of consciousness

The majority of the time we function under the *Skill-Based level of performance*. This performance level consists predominately at the automatic level. We have subconscious input that is processed using memorized sets of actions. Our brain takes in this subconscious sensory input, analyzes it into the most probable construct based on past experience and produces a subconscious action (Heuristics). We see the normal traffic pattern on our typical way to work. We start the car, pull out of the drive, use the gas, brakes, turn signals, steering wheel with very little thought. This process is fast and reasonably accurate (but not completely).

When a new variable opens up for us, we move into the *Rule-Based Level of performance*. This forces us temporarily out of the "ozone" and into reality (semi-consciousness) for brief periods of time. Someone pulls in front of us, traffic slows down, a traffic alert overhead, etc., causing us to wake up and adjust into a semiconscious area. We still use prior rules and behavior learned previously but we are not required to stay there for long. We go back to listening to the radio, pushing the gas pedal, occasionally looking in the mirror, etc.

Sudden changes, especially when these are unexpected or in our distant memory, force us into alertness (consciousness). We may attempt to solve these using skill-based or rule-based behaviors, but this is unsuccessful so we need to process and perform using *Knowledge-based* skill sets.

Someone slams on their brakes ahead or some obstacle appears and traffic comes to a halt. We need to wake up and determine what to do next (sit and wait, look for an alternate route, get out of the way of emergency vehicles, etc.). The real problems come in if we mentally do not accept that the situation has changed and remain in lower levels of function.

> This may or may not be effective depending on the level of change, the level of threat, the need to rapidly make alternate decisions. We probably will end up with erroneous analysis of the situation leading to an erroneous action. The skill-based and rule-based performance levels are typically very fast but do not provide what we need when something is unexpected and new to us. Unfortunately, knowledge-based behavior is slow and typically cannot keep up with these scenarios. Solutions? Yes, we train for these types of scenarios using knowledge-based behavior until they become skill-based.
>
> Adapted from Reason, J., Managing the Risks of Organizational Accidents. Burlington VT: Ashgate, 1997. [53]

While a *positive attribute* may be that this process works quickly and relatively effectively, on the *negative side*, it potentially can provide faulty solutions. That is, defects in the output can arise as a result of errors at any point in the sequence of input interpretation. [58, 64-68]

Reason clearly summarized the potential pitfalls in this processing, as "*the price we pay for this automatic processing of information is that perceptions, memories, thoughts, and actions have a tendency to err in the direction of the familiar and expected.*" [65]

Optical illusions are classic examples of how this process can work quickly but can also be deceiving. One early example of how our mind simply fills in the blanks in its attempt to be fast and efficient, is the 'Kanizsa' triangle, named for Gaetano Kanizsa (died 1993), who published his findings in 1955. (Figure 7) [69]

When we look at the three figures we automatically visualize a white triangle. This triangle itself does not exist, but we persistently see a white triangle that is brighter than the surrounding white area. [68]

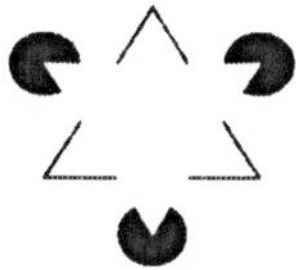

Figure 7 Gaetano Kanizsa triangle

Kanizsa, G. Margini quasi-percettivi in campi con stimolazione omogenea. *Rivista di Psicologia.* 1955;49(1):7–30. [69]

As Laurence Gonzales and many others remind us, while heuristics improves our performance in many scenarios and allows us to be more efficient and not strain on the routine environmental stimuli surrounding us, it can prove to be deadly if we don't take the time to analyze the situation in front of us especially in times of a crisis. Gonzales explains that "mental models can become stable, even in the face of clear information that would seem to contradict them, leading us into deteriorating conditions, ignoring obvious hazards.

"Our biggest enemy is often our own vision of the world. All of us carry the baggage of past assumptions called 'mental models,' which can affect our actions and how we view our surroundings. The ability to shake free of these models and gain new perspectives is what separates victims from survivors—in the wilderness, business, and relationships."

When we see, touch, smell, or hear something we automatically attempt to convert that image into something we are familiar with. Unfortunately, if we have never encountered that exact stimulus previously, we tend to find something else we are more comfortable associating with.

This process is even more ingrained when we are tired or distracted. To avoid this, if we know we are tired or distracted, we have to focus on every stimulus to assure we are processing it correctly. [62, 70]

Confirmation Bias and Fixation: "This square peg *is* going to fit into that round hole!"

Another problem we encounter is when our mind, based on past experience, creates an image where such an image does not really exist. It is as though once we commit to a judgment, any contradictory evidence is discounted in favor of any confirmatory evidence. *Once our mind has made up its mind it is not going to change its mind!* This is not a character flaw, since cognitive biases seem to be a normal feature in the way humans reason. [72, 73]

Once our mind has made up its mind
it is not going to change its mind!

Following a fatal encounter by an experienced anesthesia team's failure to call for a surgical airway after multiple unsuccessful intubation attempts, Fioratou's group designed an experimental study to help explain confirmation or fixation bias. In their necklace link study, participants were asked to join four groups of chains each three links long, but using only three moves of breaking and reconnecting the chains. Ninety-seven percent of respondents could not perform this act because they were *fixated* on their ultimate goal to guide their path towards completion of the task. That is, they were fixed on the ultimate goal of joining the four chains and would never consider breaking any. See Figure 3, page 293 for a diagram of this experiment.

They termed this "hill-climbing heuristics." That is, we select moves that reduce the distance between the current state and the goal state. We avoid any moves that seem to take us backwards, such as breaking one of the chains of three links and using those three individual links to join the remaining three chains to make a single chain of twelve links in only three open-closing moves. [74] As noted in Figure 8, page 94, this is a reminder of why we focus on the wrong goals in crisis situations, such as emergency airway scenarios.

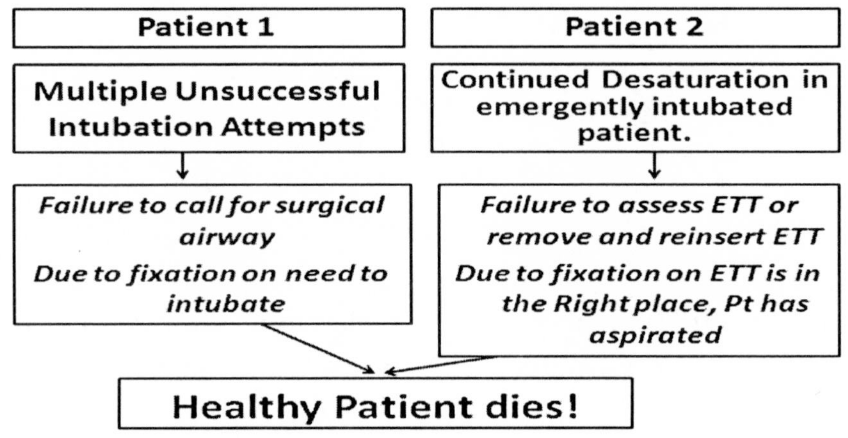

Figure 8 Fixation—Confirmation Bias Errors resulting in failed resolution of an airway problem.

Dynamic System Responses—Oversteering: "Whoa, there! Slow down a bit!"

As Dörner describes, "The tendency to over steer is characteristic of human interaction in dynamic systems," meaning that we all too often let ourselves be guided by the situation at each stage and then try to regulate the situation.

This is similar to what happens when the average person drives off the shoulder and instinctively flings the car back into the path of other cars. The goal is to get back onto the freeway, but the usual startle response heightens that goal, instinctively causing most to overreact and oversteer in the direction they want to go.

We simply apply overdoses of established measures and make the situation worse, as in when one gets lost in the wilderness. As panic sets in, the tendency is to continue to try to make ones way to the point of origin and wander around as one becomes even more lost. [23]

It is rare for a lost hiker (or surgeon) to simply *stop* and go back to where they last knew where they were or to simply quit and wait for help. *But* that is what one needs to do when they find they are lost—*stop and seek help.* [75,76]

Mental Mistakes through Complacency and Familiarity: "Eh? Don't worry about it!"

Just like seat belts and safer vehicles promote risky driving habits, [77] James Reason stated almost two decades ago that "almost every day we choose whether or not to cut corners in order to meet operational demands. For the most part, such shortcuts bring no bad effects and so become a habitual part of routine work practices. It's easy to forget to fear things that rarely happen. Unfortunately, this gradual reduction in the systems safety margins exposes it to increasingly vulnerable accident-causing factors." [53]

Clearly, once teams accept potential risky behavior in their environment based on prior acceptable outcome experience, even if that act is known to be dangerous, it is virtually impossible to negate that behavior thereafter. Refer to section "What is Human Error?" above for many examples of complacency and cutting corners in aviation.

Similarly, it is human nature to enter a deep store of skill-based performance when executing functions that are routine (familiar) to them. Wilderness rescue literature is laden with examples of "the vacation state of mind." These consist of a) poor preparation, b) lack of alertness, and c) loss of Situational Awareness (to be described below) when one enters a realm of familiarity.

The majority of surgical procedures are undertaken with a mindset that everything will be routine with relatively little chance of unexpected events. This is a common pattern seen in the etiology of wilderness and many other accidents; that is, the victim was not expecting and hence not prepared for a sudden life-threatening event.

Daniel Kahneman explains in his book why this is so. It turns out that when we are in a happy and loose mood we tend to let our guard down. We may be more creative and intuitive but also less vigilant and prone to error. We are lazy. When we are sad or tense we are more suspicious, analytical, and tend to put in more effort.

It seems counterintuitive that we would miss analytical challenges when not under stress, but in fact that is when we are less likely to double check our solutions. When we are in a good mood, there is no threat, but when we are in a bad mood, we not at "cognitive ease" and therefore want more control over our environment.

The same can be said to be true for "jumping to a conclusion." Taking a short supply of information and making a conclusion quickly without much further assessment is efficient in many circumstances. If the threat is low this saves time and effort. If the situation is unfamiliar and more threatening, then jumping to a conclusion can potentially be deadly.

For fun ask someone who is relaxed this question, "How many animals of each kind did Moses take onto the ark?" Don't be surprised if those, whose guard is down, totally miss the illogical aspect of this question. If you are bold, try this on a less-relaxed subject and see they most likely will put more thought into it. [62]

Vacation State of Mind

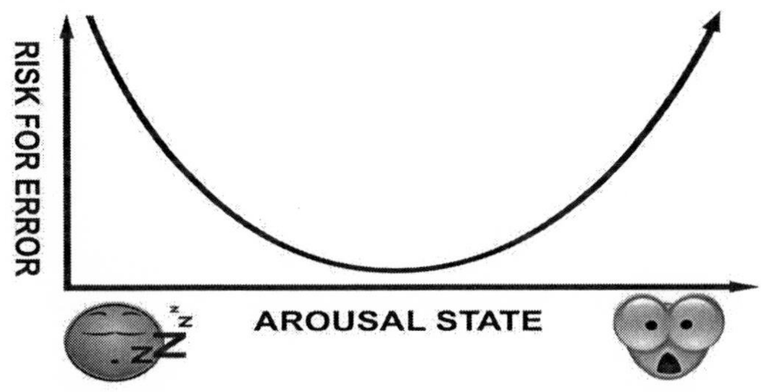

Figure 9 Vacation State of Mind: Risk for error based on arousal state. According to Daniel Kahneman, your risk for making an error is heightened when you are overly relaxed (lazy) and overly stressed or panicked. When you are highly aroused, you tend to be more focused and suspicious.

Adapted with permission from: Kahneman D. *Thinking Fast and Slow*. New York, NY: Farrar, Straus and Giroux; 2011. [62]

Wilderness Accident Similarities

It is often stated that the majority of wilderness accidents share one of the common traits found in Figure 10 [70, 71, 78-80]

This can also be said to be true for misadventures in surgical care as well. Many of these simple mistakes hinge upon being overly complacent in our approach to a procedure. As in wilderness accidents, this may be due to our being familiar with this procedure we have performed on a frequent basis, to insufficient information gathering which otherwise would have heightened our alertness or to distractions diverting our attention away from potential warning signs we missed.

Summit Hypnosis, False optimism, Over-Commitment	Refusal to quit / turn back, in spite of recognized hazards, due to focus on "summit" and ignoring dangers; frequently due to significant planning or expenses

Poor planning	Failure to imagine a worse-case scenario and planning for it; not having a bail-out plan
Poor conditioning	Failure to know one's limits; Overestimating one's ability
Inattentiveness	Due to distractions, being preoccupied or lethargy due to lack of sleep, illness, or substances
Loss of common sense	Ignoring known safety precautions
Poor or no communication	Failure to verify that leaders are as good as they say they are
Expert Halo	Trusting someone who proclaims to be or self-validates as an expert with minimal or no validation, in spite of obvious dangers or straying from known precautions
Conformity, Familiarity	Doing something risky because it has "always been done that way," the route has been a matter of routine for some time, or because someone else is doing it that way so it must be ok
Going solo	Heading out into a difficult area w/ no backup, no partner; or not communicating an itinerary with anyone
Ignoring the weather forecast	Not heeding known warnings

Figure 10 Deadly Sins: Shared Traits of Wilderness Victims
70, 71, 78-80

Situational Awareness (Common Sense), Keep Your Head Up! "Hey, did you see that?! Where did *that* come from?!"

Situation awareness (SA) simply put is knowing what is going on around you *and* knowing what is important based on the operator's occupational goals and decision task. (See section C, "Crisis Management" below for details surrounding generalized surgeon decision analysis process).

This is a continual process that starts with the perception of elements in the environment followed by the comprehension of the current situation. According to Mica Endsley (chief scientist US Air Force Pentagon) (via personal communication) 88% of aviation accidents involving human error were associated with poor SA. Seventy-six percent of SA errors occur in pilots due to *problems in perception of needed information*, secondary to either failure in the system or cognitive processes. Comprehension involves the integration of multiple pieces of information and a determination of relevance to the person's goals. Twenty percent of SA errors occur at the *level of comprehension*. The final stage of SA is the *projection of this information into a forecast of future events and dynamics*. SA alone will not guarantee the correct strategy choice. It is possible to have total awareness of the situation, but make a wrong decision based on that information. In a review of aircraft accidents, 26.6% involved poor decision making in spite of obvious appropriate awareness of the situation. In turn it is possible to be lucky and make a great decision in spite of being totally unaware of the situation surrounding you. This cannot be a passive process whereby one receives information yet is not actively involved. After information is processed, the recipient must act upon this in whatever role they are expected to have in a given situation. [81]

Fatigue, Environmental Stressors, and Distractions: "Hey! Can you keep it down a bit?"

Fatigue, burnout, and environmental stressors are underrated, under-investigated causes of human distraction. In spite of volumes of research on environmental stressors in other complex industries, the medical field has developed scant research on stress and distraction on surgeons and the surgical team (most of this has been in the past few recent years).

Balch et al. related that burnout and other measures of surgeon distress correlate directly with increasing work hours over eighty hours a week and nights on call over twice a week among American surgeons. They noted that "when physicians are in distress, their performance in delivering care can be suboptimal" which increases risk for a home-work conflict and lapse in judgment. [82]

Moorthy et al studied the effects of stressors on surgeons in a study assessing the impairment of dexterity and incidence of errors after subjecting surgeons to three stressors: a simple verbal mathematical task, operating theatre background noise at 80 to 85 dB, and performance as quickly as possible. A significantly higher number of errors occurred as measured by a significant increase in the path length per movement of their hands, under all four stress-inducing conditions (the prior ones individually or combined) compared to quietness. [83]

Finally, Feuerbacher's recent publication concluded that "Younger, less-experienced surgeons are more prone to distraction in the O.R.—and to make surgical errors as a result, and participants facing disruptions did much worse in the afternoons, although conventional fatigue didn't appear to be an issue." During simulated laparoscopic cholecystectomy, surgeons were distracted by noises, questions, conversation, or other commotion in the operating room. While the young surgeons, aged 27 to 35, were trying to perform the lap cholecystectomy, a cell phone would ring, followed later by a metal tray clanging to the floor. Questions would be posed about problems developing with a previous surgical patient—a necessary conversation—and someone off to the side would begin talking about politics, a not-so-necessary but fairly realistic distraction. Interrupting questions caused the most major errors (such as damage to internal organs, ducts, and arteries), followed by sidebar conversations. [84]

Interruptions due to cell phones, pagers, side-bar conversations, direct questions, clanging trays, wrong instruments and so on create distractions potentially resulting in adverse events.
Reducing distractions reduces mistakes!

Another study at the Mayo Clinic in cardiothoracic surgery found that surgical errors increased significantly with increases in flow disruptions. Flow disruptions consisted of communication failures, equipment and technology problems, extraneous interruptions, training-related distractions, and issues in resource accessibility, with teamwork-communication failures being the strongest predictor. [85]

While this scant research regarding stress and distraction among surgeons is commendable, it barely scratches the surface on what is necessary for the health care industry to understand how stress and distraction influence adverse outcomes. Furthermore, this focuses only on surgeons, with no focus on the surgical team as a whole where distraction and stress, especially in a crisis situation, are not uncommon. As expected, these effects of distraction are magnified significantly during the stress-panic responses that will be described in detail later.

Is There Any Hope for Us? Can We Prepare Ourselves to Prevent these Mental Errors in the O.R.?

Inevitably as one considers the various mental miscues that would allow a surgeon to make a mistake which results in damage to the common bile duct during cholecystectomy or the right middle lobe bronchus during a right lower lobectomy (Figure 11), we need to assure that we take precautions to draw attention to these structures during these procedures. According to Dr. Way and others, keeping a mental check sheet and stop points to prevent the procedures from simply being a routine will assist the surgeon in keeping alert and avoid these missteps.

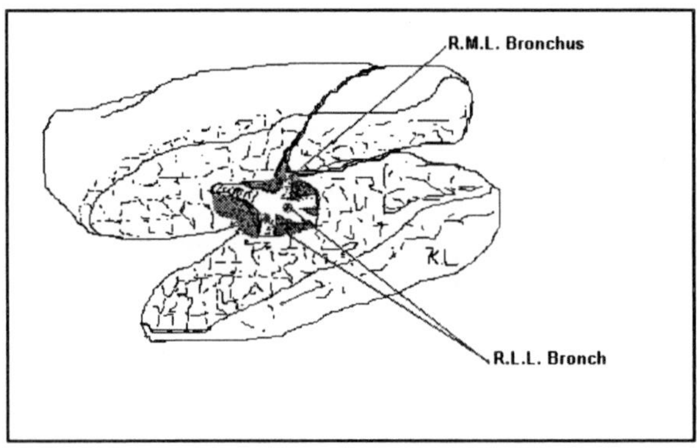

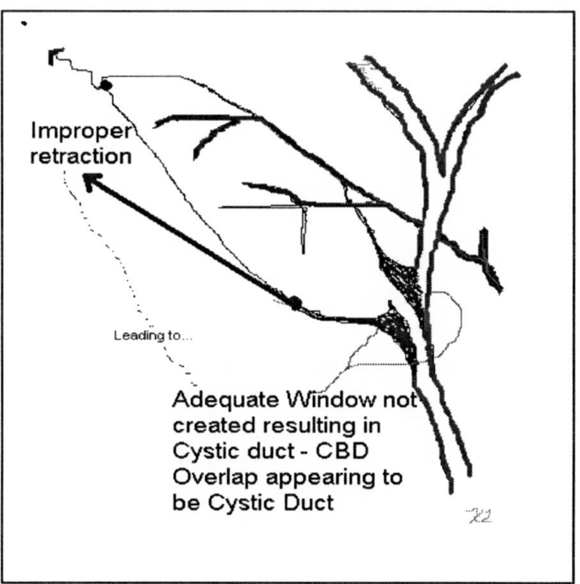

Figure 11 a, b Potential junctures in surgical procedures where cognitive error has greatest risk.

a. During a lung right lower lobectomy, the middle lobe bronchus is prone to inadvertent ligation due to unawareness, distraction, or heuristic tendencies of the surgeon.
b. During a routine laparoscopic cholecystectomy, the common bile duct is prone to injury due to poor landmark exposure, distraction, or heuristic tendencies of the surgeon.

For example, during laparoscopic cholecystectomy, simple things such as keeping mental awareness to widely open the hepatocystic triangle (aka a critical view), retracting the infundibulum inferiorly-anteriorly and the fundus up towards the diaphragm, move infundibulum back and forth (waving the flag, to see both sides), validate critical view of safety before clipping/dividing structures, making sure clips are all the way across the duct and remember *if the duct is wider than the clips*, think twice. [58]

Can Anything Be Done to Stop This Mess?

As noted above, heuristic influences on cognitive error are heightened when the new paradigm is unfamiliar. This is augmented further when the victim has a lapse in consciousness due to fatigue or distraction. Having said that, by this point it should be obvious that one of the simplest steps in cognitive error reduction should begin with *reductions in distractions* especially during crucial points in the care of the patient.

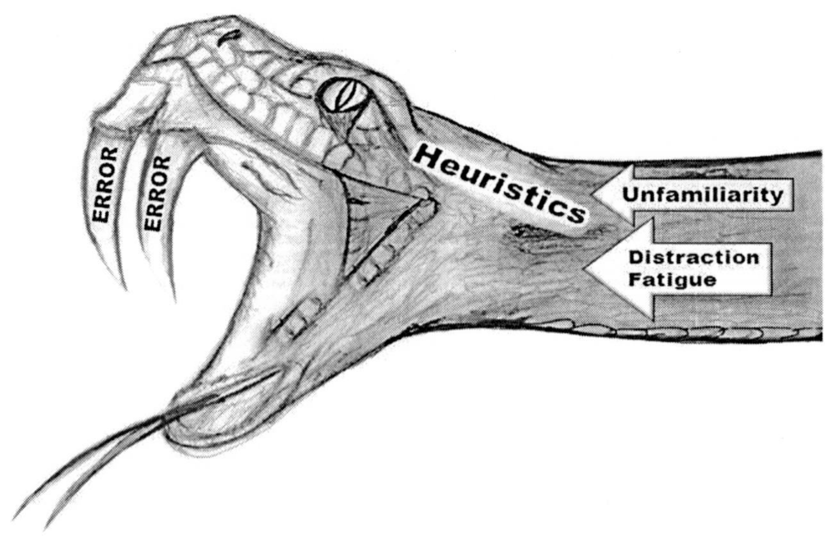

Figure 12 Influences that increase our susceptibility to Heuristic tendencies: in addition to our state of arousal, our tendency to fall prey to prior modeling to sensory input is drastically augmented if we are unfamiliar with that stimulus or we are victim to lapses of consciousness (fatigue or distraction). [70, 71, 85- 88]

Weick and Sutcliffe use the term *mindfulness* to describe "strengthening the capabilities to hold onto an object being perceived." Any method that prevents the mind from wandering away from the task at hand assists in strengthening that mindfulness. They describe a Navy Admiral who insisted that mistakes are not intentional, but due to distraction. Furthermore he encouraged routine tracking of distractions and reporting to the crew to enhance awareness.

Additionally, we have to learn to detect when we are being distracted or fatigued and pay closer attention to the stimuli around us and focus on whether those are indeed familiar or in actuality unrecognized input that we must process to a greater degree. Distractions and fatigue are just a single part of systems issues to be detailed later. [88]

Maladaptive Stress Response Reversal Training

While a minority of us seem to be naturally gifted to handle a survival situation (traits described below), the majority of us simply have to learn to train to adapt contrary to our normal behavior. Training people to respond to stress in an appropriate manner is extremely difficult if they are not provided background information as to why they responded in that manner in the first place. This will be explained further below.

Reduce Interruptions
Reduce Distractions
Improve Communication
Increase Stop Points at Critical Parts of Case
Train Your Team!

Simple methods to assist in the reduction of cognitive errors during any procedure

PART TWO

System's Role in Error Mitigation

System's Role in the Mitigation of a Single Human Cognitive Error Preventing Propagation into an Operating Room Crisis

It's Not Who Cut the Cheese, but How You Sliced It

> "Every accident, of any kind, is preceded by a chain of events or errors, but each is set into motion at one irreversible moment. Until that moment the accident might have been prevented."
>
> Jill Fredston, *Snowstruck: In the Grip of Avalanches, 2005,* Mariner Books, Seattle

History of Systems Theory: Human Error Did This! Cause or Symptom?

Two basic theories on the evolution of disasters were presented above:

1. Bad-Apple Theory
2. Systems Theory

The "Bad-Apple Theory" assumes that "human error causes bad accidents; failures are unpleasant, unsuspected surprises and complex systems are basically safe." Multiple causes of "accidental" human error were described above.

"Systems Theory" concludes that in complex systems "errors are inevitable products of people doing the best they can in systems that contain multiple subtle vulnerabilities and that errors are symptoms of deeper troubles." [28] One of the better descriptions of this relationship was by J. Calland in 2002: "Events, objects, locations, and methods do not exist independently, but rather are *intertwined* as interdependent components of complex systems. Complex systems also incorporate *multiple layers* of seemingly unrelated issues, including social, legal, cultural, and economic factors, which ultimately shape the system's final form. If an alteration occurs in any one of the components making up a complex system, its effect ripples throughout the entire system." [18]

Reason contended that people are always too quick to blame human error as a cause of an organizational accident rather than acknowledge the error may have been a consequence of organizational failure. It is assumed that people are regarded as free agents and their errors are voluntary actions. While in some cases people can behave carelessly, a careless act does not necessarily make the person stupid or careless. Evidence, from a large number of accident investigations has indicated that these incidents are more likely a consequence of error-prone situations and activities rather than error-prone workers. A significant discussion on Reason's theory of organizational accidents will follow soon. [53]

Dekker stated clearly that human error is not the cause of failure, but it is a symptom of organizational failure. Assessments of safety concerns are hindered by hindsight (outcome) bias where the assessors are interpreting the situation after the outcome is known and no one is looking at local rationality. [89]

People do what makes sense in their current circumstances.

Because of these misconceptions, no relationship was paid to the interaction of individual components leading to disasters in complex systems until after three independent, but scenario-related disasters occurred across the globe in the 1970s.

These awareness-provoking incidents were:

1. The KLM 747 - Pan Am 747 disaster of March 27 1977 at Los Rodeos Airport, Tenerife Island, Canary Islands
2. United Airlines Flight 173 Crash in Portland Oregon, December 28, 1978
3. The Three-Mile Island Accident of Dauphin County Pennsylvania, March 28 1979

Shortly after the Three-Mile Island disaster, Perrow provided an eye-opening description of the entity of *normal* accidents. He stated that some systems are so complex, accidents are bound to happen. In these systems, processes happen so fast, they cannot be turned off in these systems. Once the process is disturbed, recovery from the initial disturbance is not possible and the negative effects will spread quickly and irretrievably for some time.

In these complex, self-organizing systems there are "numerous agents acting in simple roles that cause actions of one or more agents to influence what others do." Subsequent to these reports, Roberts, Rochlin, and LaPorte at Berkley described the operations on the carrier *Carl Vinson* 1987, as a HIGH RELIABILITY ORGANIZATION (HRO). [90] HRO's are organizations that consistently avoid catastrophes in an environment where "normal" accidents can be predicted due to the complexity of the system. [91]

In 1990, James Reason described the Cumulative Act Effect whereby the majority of accidents can be traced from one to four levels of failure:

1. Organizational influences: from organizational management, time pressure, output pressure, governmental pressure, etc.
2. Unsafe supervision: organizational front line management
3. Preconditions for unsafe acts, the "Dirty Dozen:" lack of communication, complacency, lack of knowledge, distraction, lack of teamwork, fatigue, lack of resources, pressure, lack of assertiveness, stress, lack of awareness and "the norms" or unwritten rules everyone follows (courtesy of Gordon Dupont, CEO, System-Safety www.system-safety.com. For a more detailed list, refer to Figure 1, page 4 of the Boeing MEDA guide) [26]
4. The unsafe acts themselves (inserting an expired implant, retained foreign body, wrong site surgery, wrong patient, transected common bile duct / ureter / right middle lobe bronchus, or failure to notice low fuel/altitude indicator, pushing wrong buttons, etc.)

It was proposed that organizations should establish defenses against these failures through identification of the weaknesses in the individual parts of the system, followed by the creation of a series of barriers of varying size and position to prevent perpetuation of that error or failure to the next level. It was identified that systemic failure would occur when all individual barrier weaknesses aligned, permitting *a trajectory of accident opportunity* so that a hazard passes through all of the holes in all the levels of defense.

Not soon thereafter, this was described as the "Swiss-Cheese concept." One alarming, yet all too familiar potential adverse event seen in the O.R. is the retention of a surgical item at the conclusion of the surgical procedure. As seen in Figure 13, there are a multitude of steps involved in the prevention of adverse events during any patient care scenario. If all safeguards are fully enforced, then failure at a single point should theoretically be prevented from progressing to an ultimate disastrous outcome. Failure of system safety nets at multiple points is typically required for any single error or external event to remain unmitigated and result in disaster.

Having said that, in a 2011 VA study of 28 Medical centers from 2003 - 2007, it was noted that there were 23 occurrences of retained surgical items after surgical procedures (number of procedures overall was not indicated). Half of these were sponges. In twelve of these cases there was a concurrence between the pre- and post-sponge counts, i.e. the counts "agreed." These false "correct" counts highlight the potential for human error in the processes involved during a sponge count. If this occurs at only one step, theoretically the retained sponge would be detected before the patient left the room, but if failure occurs at every step, then the patient has a potential for leaving the O.R. with a sponge retained in the patient's body. [92]

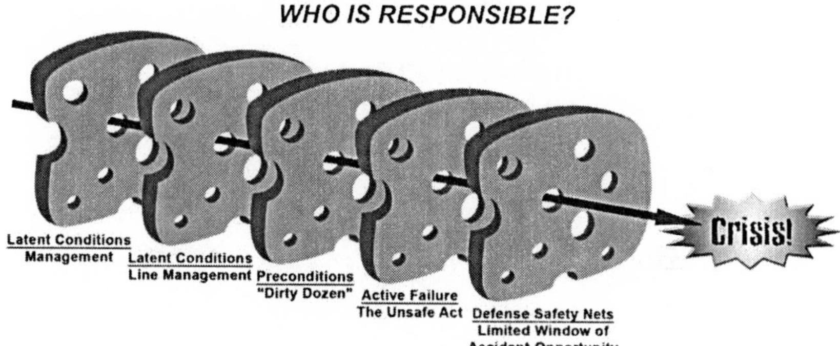

Figure 13 Adaptation of James Reason's Stages in the Development of an Organizational Accident:

Latent conditions—upper level management decisions or lack of decisions on important matters that have downstream effects (such as budget cuts, hiring deficits, training deficits, production pressure, lack of correction of communication or behavior deficits, etc.). Under Boeing MEDA (Maintenance Error Decision Aid) Management, proactivity should eliminate 80-90% of the risk for error in the field.

Active failures are the unsafe actions done by the worker, pilot, tech, etc.

Preconditions are conditions that are known but not addressed in the organization that predispose workers to an active failure. Human factors training can eliminate the majority of these.

Adapted from Gordon Dupont, CEO Systems Safety (at www.system-safety.com) and Reason JT, Managing the Risks of Organizational Accidents, 1997 [53]

Figure 13 brings the pieces of the organizational accident together. According to the FAA, Boeing MEDA, 80 - 90% of contributing factors to errors/violations are under management control, while the remaining 10-20% under the control of the front line technicians.

In reality only 10-20% of errors are amenable to human factor training to eliminate preconditions. Upper level and supervisory management can make changes to reduce or eliminate the majority of contributing factors to an error or violation, reducing the probability of future events. [26, 65]

TICKING TIME BOMB
Preconditions
Gaps in: Knowledge, communication, awareness, teamwork with complacency, stress, fatigue...
Increases in:
Production Pressures
New Hires
Staff Work Pressure
Equipment Failure
Corner Cutting
Lapses/Missteps
Reductions in:
Funding
Supplies
Support Staff
Equipment Repair
DISASTER

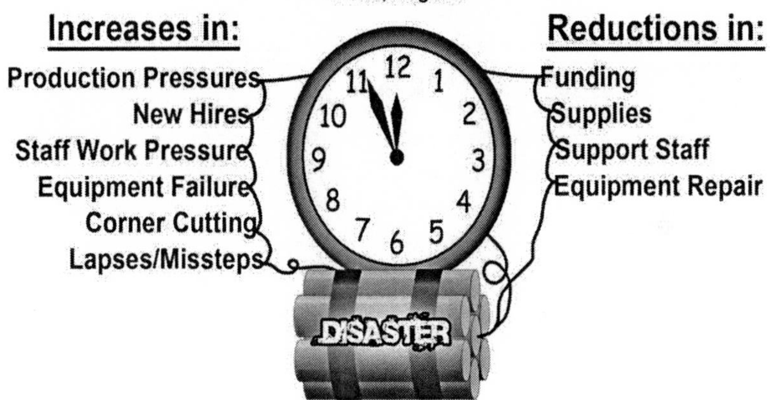

Figure 14 Ticking Time Bomb: How everything in the organization is interconnected but seemingly hidden till everything times itself perfectly at the instant the disaster occurs. Lapses, missteps, slips, corner cuts seem to be preceded by equipment failures and supply reductions which were preceded by multiple preconditions, seemingly brought about by short staffing in equipment repair and supply services, compounded by new poorly trained hires and increased workload brought about by staffing shortages that came about by budget cuts and production increase pressures.

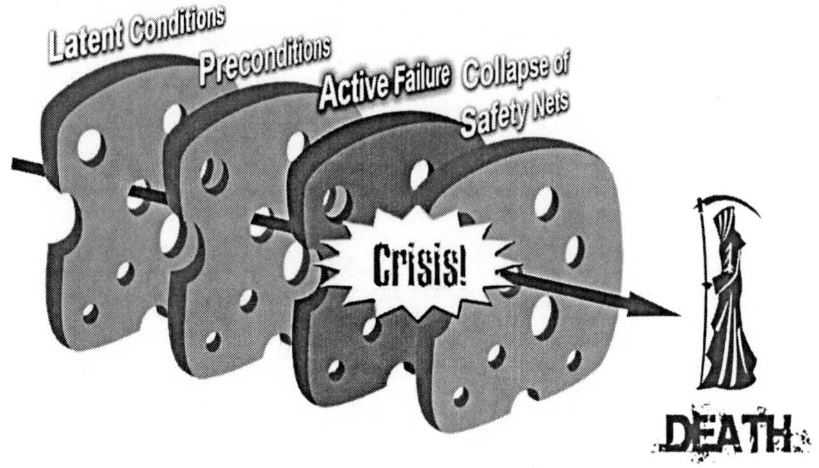

Figure 15 Use of Reason's System Model to explain transition from a difficult procedure to a crisis (misadventure or other unexpected event) to a disaster (death in the O.R.).

Latent conditions are brought about by administrative pressure to do more cases, lack of ability to transfer difficult cases to higher level center, recent release of staff or hiring of cheaper, less experienced staff.

Preconditions exist for years and include fatigue, stress, ambivalence, lack of knowledge, reduction in resources followed by teamwork and communication degradation.

System Safety nets are then discovered to be absent leading to propagation of a misadventure or other unexpected event into a patient care disaster. Safety nets typically revolve around lack of resources thought to exist but in actuality are absent (staff, training, supplies, equipment, etc.) as well as distractions created by inefficiencies elsewhere in the organization.

Crew Resource Management and Medical Team Training—"Checklists and Acronyms! You gotta be kidding me! Do any of these work?"

In 1979, in response to the 1977 Tenerife Island Airport disaster and the 1978 United Airlines disaster, NASA created a workshop titled "Resource Management on the Flight Deck," examining the role that human error plays in air catastrophes. Their conclusion of this and of subsequent reports was that human error caused or contributed to over 50% of aviation accidents. At least 70% of human error mishaps were connected with aircrew factors, and 56% of these resulted from at least one resource management failure.

In "an analysis of 35,000 reports of incidents over 7.5 years, almost 50% resulted from a flight crew error, and an additional 35% were attributed to air traffic controller error." The bottom line was that root cause analyses by safety experts found that errors frequently occurred *because flight crews fail to effectively manage the resources available to them* (e.g., fail to verify information when uncertain about it, fail to plan for contingencies). [24, 93]

In response to the United Airlines crash of 1978, the National Transportation Safety Board (NTSB) singled out the following causal factors to that and other airline crashes:

- Captain's failure to accept input from junior crew members (wrong stuff)
- Lack of assertiveness of flight engineers [25]

In 1981, United Airlines hired consultants experienced in developing training programs for corporations trying to enhance managerial effectiveness. Their program was modeled after managerial grid training developed by psychologists Blake and Mouton (1964). They modified this to address both the lack of assertiveness by juniors and the authoritarian behavior of captains through changing individual styles and correcting deficiencies in individual behavior. [94]

In response to the NASA workshop report and the United Airlines consultative report, structured training courses titled "Crew Resource Management" (CRM) were instituted. CRM was the process of training crews to reduce pilot error by making better use of the human resources on the flight deck. CRM emphasizes the role of human factors in high-stress, high-risk environments. The organizers of the course defined CRM as "using all available sources—information, equipment, and people—to achieve safe and efficient flight operations." This was accomplished through focus on team training, simulation, interactive group debriefings, and measurement and improvement of aircrew performance. [25]

Crew Resource Management

Focus on:

1. Team training
2. Simulation
3. Interactive group debriefings
4. Measurement and improvement of aircrew performance

One decade after United Airlines developed their Crew Resource Management training program, Alan Diehl, a world renowned aviation safety investigator, presented a seminar at the International Society of Air Safety investigators. Surprisingly, after ten years of effective CRM institutionalization, many aviation leaders were not completely convinced they had enough data to mandate CRM across the board. One decade later controversy and naysayers persisted.

In his report, Diehl reviewed the results of 28 NTSB reviewed accidents and 169 US Air force accidents from 1987-89. His conclusion was that 24 of the 28 NTSB and 113-169 US Air Force accidents involved aircrew error and that Cockpit Management training was responsible for reduction of 36 - 86% of accidents in the pilot groups trained. [27]

As noted in many institutions, CRM is called for as a leadership reactionary response after an *event* occurs. For team training to be effective, it has to be taught *proactively and* as an ongoing learning experience, *not* retrospectively after a disaster.

In my mind, two 2009 airline crashes symbolize the effects when a) CRM standards are adhered to, and b) when they are ignored. In one crash the crew acted in exemplary fashion, utilizing the positive effects of CRM. In the other, systems management principles clearly failed due to "bad apples" when the crew ignored basic safety standards.

The January 15, 2009 crash of US Airways Flight 1549 into the Hudson River, after an encounter with geese, shows how crew training can yield high quality team management skills and save the lives of passengers on an aircraft that was on an otherwise fatal course. Flight 1549 successfully landed into the Hudson River and, due to the reliability of crew performance, all 155 occupants left the plane alive.

The Colgan Air flight 3407 crash in Buffalo in February 12, 2009, reveals the fatal consequences when pilots fail to follow standard cockpit principles and become complacent in their required monitoring of their airspeed indicators. Ignoring standard safe approach precautions, known as the *sterile cockpit,* which prohibits nonessential conversation within the cockpit during critical phases of flight, the pilots chatted about personal matters without attention to their airspeed, failing to note the low-speed cue resulting in a stall which was not properly responded to by the crew. All 49 occupants died just 5 miles short of the Buffalo airport. [95,96]

Surprisingly, it was not until 2004 that the first reports began to circulate regarding the merits of CRM and its acceptance of its application in Medicine. Medical Team Training (MTT) quickly became the synonym of CRM in the medical field. [97]

Simultaneously, as noted above, while there was heightened focus on the medical field's rate of adverse events, The Joint Commission developed their "Universal Protocol to prevent confusions in surgical procedures that had been resulting in wrong site/side surgery." [13] Finally, the evolution of perioperative checklists, similar to those used in the flight industry was beginning.

Initial studies prior to 2009 did not show much positive effect from Medical Team training, but studies from 2010 and on have steadily shown benefit to these on mortality, mistakes and overall team function. CRM/MTT effects deteriorate with time and training individual teams alone frequently does not suffice. [98-109]

As noted in Figure 16, there are some similarities and some differences between team dynamics in the cockpit and in the Operating Room. The similarities allow checklists and team training to partially carry over to the operating room but there are some differences that prevent these aviation models from completely eliminating errors and crises in the operating room. For the most part, when O.R. procedures proceed according to expected pathways, checklists similar to those used in the cockpit work well to assure we do not make a mistake. That is, the checklists work according to plan when there is no urgency or threat. That benefit seems to be lost as soon as a crisis occurs when the unknown becomes a factor.

Similar problems are seen in the fire service when an unexpected event arises and there are many unknowns that have to be dealt with simultaneously. It appears that crises in firefighting arise because fires, like humans, are unpredictable at best during a crisis. Checklists work well after the situation has been controlled and the team comprehends the majority of the factors involved in the crisis. In the firefighting field, jumping to conclusions and reacting rapidly without taking a few seconds to assimilate information can be deadly. This is also true in O.R. crises, where jumping to conclusions without adequate communication and information sharing can be detrimental if not lethal for the patient. [25, 111-117]

Similarities and Differences between a Cockpit and an Operating Room

Standard Operating Procedures: Rules and Regulations

Cockpit	Operating Room
Conducts a flight in accordance with clear rules and regulations. Pilot's tasks are directed by Standard Operating Procedures and a variety of checklists and manuals, dictating actions in normal and emergency situations.	Standardized regulations, SOP's, and Checklists are in the early stages, not well accepted by all, and remain variable to institution. Checklists have proven more beneficial for use in Human-Machine interfaces especially in times of crisis.

Interaction with Other Groups

Cockpit	Operating Room
Although the flight crew must interact with other groups in the the system, their primary work-place is clearly defined and isolated.	The Operating Room has many subgroups, is much more fluid and dynamic. It is without formalized control mechanisms.

Team Size

Cockpit	Operating Room
A small team working for the same organization. Commercial Teams have all received the same training, but may not have worked with one another. Once the mission is underway, the team stays together until it is complete.	A team that changes construct on a month-to-month, day-to-day basis. Typically all work with one another on a daily basis but construct may change during the case. The team membership at the beginning of the mission may vary during the mission.

Complexity

Cockpit	Operating Room
Complex. While clearly defined, there are opportunities for variation in the combined influences of weather, air-traffic and mechanical problems. These require a variety of decision making processes and prioritization among alternatives.	The Operating Room is a much more complex environment psychologically than the cockpit.

Human Error as a Cause of Accidents

Cockpit

Research into causes of air disasters in the late 1970s led investigators to the disturbing conclusion that more than 70% of air crashes involved human error rather than mechanical failure or weather.

Operating Room

Investigation of incidents in anesthesia suggest that 75 - 80% include human error, including failures in communication, decision making, interpersonal conflict, and lack of teamwork. In a survey of anesthesiologists, 24% admitted committing a fatal error.

Training, Research, and Information Sharing

Cockpit

In aviation, everyone shares a concern with safety. Organizations are open to research that has the potential to decrease the likelihood of accidents. Research in aviation is facilitated by archival data available from accident investigations and incident reports. Regular training and performance evaluation of flight crews in simulators and aircraft are required.

Operating Room

Aviation and medicine differ greatly in their acceptance of the type of research into group behavior. Medical practice is driven by fear of litigation should evidence of substandard practice be revealed. There is also no corporate willingness to share data. Psychological training seen in pilots is rare in medicine.

Figure 16 Similarities and Differences between a Cockpit and an Operating Room [25, 110, 111, 114-117]

Poor Communication!

Communication Error: "Hey! Are you listening to me? Did you hear what I just said?"

While improvements were noted in various publications, we have not reached the point of 100% elimination for preventable adverse events in the O.R. In the end, the question still remains: "Why have CRM/MTT and perioperative checklists not persistently created a completely safe environment?"

According to the Joint Commission Center for Transforming Healthcare the causes of wrong site surgery can be found in this long list:

1. Distractions/rushing
2. Too many forms/fields
3. Someone other than the surgeon marks the site
4. Surgeon did not mark site in pre-op area.
5. Site marked not on the incision/procedure area
6. Inconsistent site marking methods
7. Documents not verified prior to patient coming to pre-op holding

8. Staff not following policy
9. Ineffective time out
10. Site not physically verified immediately before the incision/procedure
11. Primary documentation not used to verify the patient, procedure or site
12. Ineffective education and communication
13. Nurses and staff do not feel empowered to speak up
14. Senior leadership not engaged
15. Quality and risk management not fully integrated into O.R. processes (teams)
16. Staff working in silos
17. Ineffective handoff between preop and O.R.
18. No objective measurements
19. No continuing improvement processes. [118]

The key contributory factor in the majority of surgical adverse events has been communication failures. The O.R. is prone to communication errors because of its complex setting, stress levels, resistance to change, cultural differences, communication styles, compounded with the O.R. environment and administration created culture and stress.

According to "Applied Strategies for the Improvement of Patient Safety" (ASIPS -2004) two-thirds of patient safety breaches have been due to communication problems. [119, 120] Symons in the UK found that "failures had many causes but two of the most common and preventable were failures in communication between staff and delays in treatment or assessment." "If the results of this study are any indicator, one can expect four to five procedural mistakes during a postoperative course. Half of these result in significant harm and the majority of failures in the *processes* of care—from giving drugs to delivering test results and giving patients instructions—were rampant. And 51% of the instances led to serious problems." Of 352 mistakes, 256 were due to *process failures.* [121]

In a review of malpractice cases failure to communicate occurred in over one-third of reviewed cases and played a role in 20% of complications. In 444 surgical malpractice claims there was a critical communication failure in 81 cases; 56% of cases involved a failure to transmit critical information to the attending surgeon. [122]

Knowledge that communication deficiencies are the key component to adverse events is crucial for teams to develop methodologies to avoid medical error creation or the perpetuation of that error to a disaster. [110, 123-125]

Refer to Part Three, Communication, pp. 201 - 205 for more information regarding communication skills.

> "I ought to have known, my advisors ought to have known, and I ought to have been told and I ought to have asked."
> *Winston Churchill, regarding the*
> *Japanese land advance over Singapore*

Order 01.09 "Ready for Sea" Implicit Communication

"Heads of departments are to report to the master if they are aware of any deficiency which is likely to cause their departments to be unready for sea in any respect at the due sailing time. In the absence of any such report, the master will assume at the due sailing time, the vessel is ready for sea in all respects."

The ***Herald of Free Enterprise*** sank within five minutes of leaving its Belgium port when the bow doors were left open and the report was not forwarded to the master, because the Seaman responsible for that report was asleep. 193 out of 500 on board died that day due to this glitch in the communications process.

Problem associated with Communication Expectations during the 1987 sinking of the ferry ***Herald of Free Enterprise:*** This type of closed inferred communication is extremely dangerous in high risk environments. Communication should always be front-loaded and very explicit (see section on communication below). We should never be assuming that something has been accomplished until we have a confirmed report that it is so.

Investigation Reports Herald of Free Enterprise, p. 12. http://www.maib.gov.uk/publications/investigation_reports/herald_of_free_enterprise/herald_of_free_enterprise_report.cfm

- "Communication is really all anyone ever gets paid for ultimately...and if you cannot effectively communicate...you will PAY...not get paid." *Doug Firebaugh*

- "Communicate, not so that you will always be understood, but so that you will always not be misunderstood!" *F. D. Roosevelt*

- "Do not write merely to be understood. Write so you cannot possibly be misunderstood."
Robert Louis Stevenson

- "How well we communicate is determined not by how well we say things but by how well we are understood."
Andrew S. Grove

- "The greatest problem in communication is the illusion that it has been accomplished."
Daniel W. Davenport

Resilience to Error in High Reliability Organizations (HROs): "Smooth sailin', just like a ship on the ocean."

Aircraft carriers operate in a continued state of readiness and safety, utilizing a crew composed of men and women virtually all less than 20 years of age. The success of these large ships in remaining safe centers around the command's preoccupation with resilience. That is, the constant thinking about potential failure, taking nothing for granted, sensitivity to all levels of operation, and commitment to being resilient.

Part of focusing on failure includes constant assessment and rehearsal for those almost never but potentially possible events. So too, should the operating room environment be completely focused on resilience. [88]

- Preoccupation with Failure
- Reluctance to Simplify
- Sensitivity to Operations

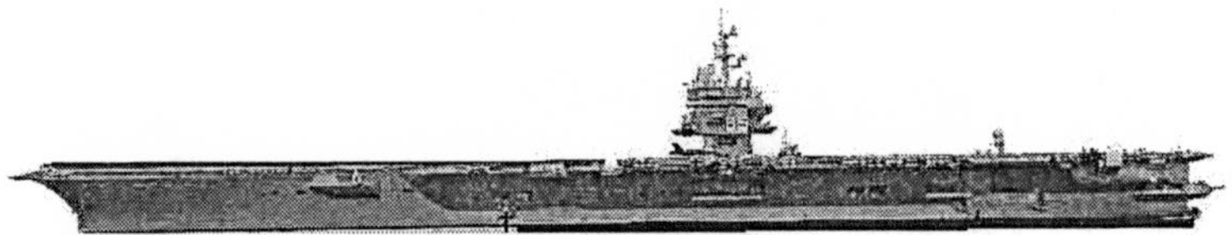

- Commitment to Resilience
- Deference to Expertise

Figure 17 HRO Principles at work on an aircraft carrier. Carriers are 1,100 by 250 feet floating cities carrying 100 aircraft and manned by 5,000 employees, the majority of which are under the age of twenty, and recently recruited by the Navy.

Adapted from: Weick KE, Sutcliffe KM. *Managing the Unexpected: Resilient Performance in an Age of Uncertainty*. San Francisco, CA: John Wiley; 2007. Photo: Lipshy KA. USS Enterprise in the James River April, 2010. [88]

"Responsibility is a unique concept. It can only reside and inhere in a single individual. You may share it with others, but your portion is not diminished. You may delegate it, but it is still with you. You may disclaim it, but you cannot divest yourself of it. Even if you do not recognize it or admit its presence, you cannot escape it. If responsibility is rightfully yours, no evasion or ignorance or passing the blame can pass the burden to someone else. Unless you can point your finger at the man responsible when something goes wrong, then you have never had anyone really responsible."

Hyman G. Rickover (1900-1986),
Director of Naval Nuclear Reactors 1949-1982

In the aftermath of the Three Mile Island accident in 1979, "Over the years, many people have asked me how I run the Naval Reactors Program, so that they might find some benefit for their own work. I am always chagrined at the tendency of people to expect that I have a simple, easy gimmick that makes my program function. Any successful program functions as an integrated whole of many factors. Trying to select one aspect as the key one will not work. Each element depends on all the others."

Hyman G. Rickover

PART THREE

Time Critical/Rapid Process Decision Making Events: Is Your Team Ready for Its Next Crisis?

Adaptive vs. Maladaptive Surgical Team Responses to an O.R. Crisis: How Team Response Can Positively or Negatively Influence the Outcome

> "The ability to deal with a crisis situation is largely dependent on the structures that have developed before chaos arrives...at a moment's notice, everything that was left unprepared becomes a complex problem, and every weakness comes rushing to the forefront."
>
> Pat Lagadec, *Preventing Chaos in a Crisis: Strategies for Prevention, Control and Damage Limitation.*
> London. McGraw-Hill 1993

"I thought you said this would make us safe! Why is my HRO not 100% error-resistant? How could that disaster have possibly happened?"

By definition, a high reliability organization is one that is so complex, it is expected that an adverse event could occur at any time, but the system is designed to minimize the effects on the rest of the system or team. The preceding section focused on the ability of an HRO to anticipate adverse events, and the need for that organization to understand the potential negative effects the staff at that organization may face. Upon anticipating these negative events, the system theoretically should have barriers established to prevent a single event from harming the organization, the team or, in a medical facility, the patient.

Paying attention to its environment and staff, and providing feedback in a meaningful manner to the teams should allow an organization to keep up with the flux as things change. But, anticipating and preparing for these events is only part of the equation. The system must be established to contain the negative event at its damage-limiting stage. After such an untoward event occurs, the team needs to have the capacity to react swiftly and control the situation.

An easy question members of an HRO probably would ask by this point in their maturity would be: *"If we have done everything to predict all the unexpected, worst-case scenarios, why should we worry?"*

The answers to that are:

- You *cannot* predict everything.
- You may not be the high reliability organization you thought you were.
- The team's preconceived notions may cloud their judgment as noted in the sections above.

In general, an unexpected disaster typically occurs when the events were totally not expected; that is, they were completely unplanned for.

There are potentially three simple forms of unexpected events:

1. Something expected does not occur.
2. An unexpected event occurs.
3. Something totally unimaginable strikes.

One must remember that just because something does not go according to plan, does not necessarily make it a disaster, and even when something does go according to plan it can result in disastrous consequences.

At the same time, having expectations about an event can create a *blind spot* as noted above during the discussion regarding Heuristics and confirmation bias. The blind spot occurs as one disconfirms evidence to the contrary of what they believed to be true. As in, "everything is just fine, it's all good." The same can be said for when the unexpected occurs: you usually know when something *unexpected* has happened because that is the moment you feel *anxious, concerned, surprised, leery…*

As noted above, it is easy at this moment to convince yourself that everything is normal, and indulge in your confirmation bias that everything is okay. As will be explained below, the sooner one recognizes the unexpected has occurred and all is *not* normal, the sooner recovery can happen. [88]

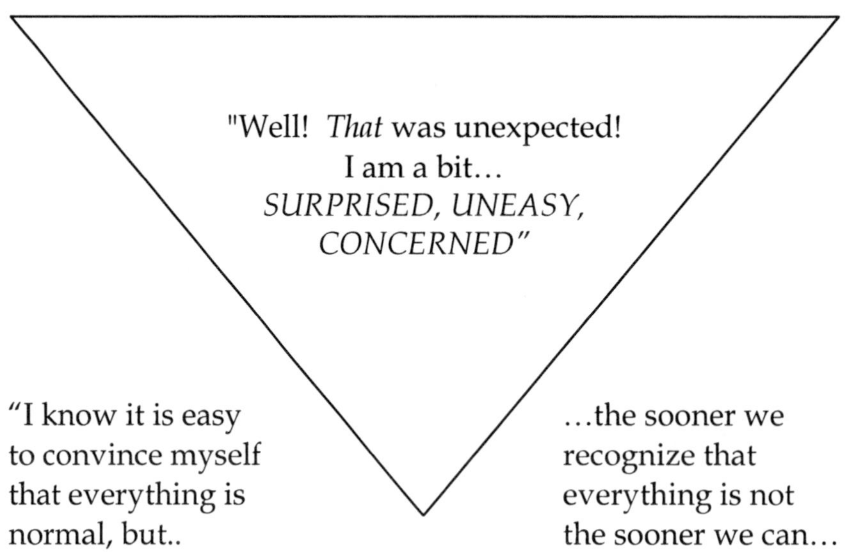

Figure 18 When one first recognizes that something unexpected arises they need to have trained themselves to

trust their instincts

rather than rely upon protective responses that try to lead them to believe all is normal.

Avoid Heuristic Confirmation / Normalcy bias, convincing you all is okay.

Adapted from: Weick KE, Sutcliffe KM. *Managing the Unexpected: Resilient Performance in an Age of Uncertainty*. San Francisco, CA: John Wiley; 2007. [88]

Knowing that it is virtually impossible to predict every significant event that can occur in an organization, the next step available would be to assess how resilient or vulnerable the team or organization is, as a whole, to an unexpected crisis.

When it comes to coping with crises in the medical field, there is little information on training the team to respond appropriately, in medical literature. The basic components for surviving a crisis or disaster would simplistically be similar in most scenarios and are found in examples from other genres of publications, especially in those dealing with wilderness survival.

It is also useful, as will be seen, for each individual to do a self-character map, to determine their own response during a crisis, because *survivors* (figuratively speaking, regarding one who responds in a productive capacity during a crisis) have a particular characteristic makeup (also to be described below) which is found in alternate resources, mostly dealing with outdoor survival. [126]

It is important to know how our negative responses to stress arise and how to develop coping mechanisms to overcome panic. It should not be surprising that *only 10 - 20% of people have the ability to stay calm in the midst of a crisis.* I can recall more than one occasion where a colleague has stated, "This patient is going to die!" or "Crap! We are never going to fix this…" and thinking to myself, "Such a catastrophic attitude in the face of adversity simply turns an upward hill climb into a formidable insurmountable obstacle." [71, 127]

Only 10 – 20% of people have the ability to stay calm in the midst of a crisis!

Crisis Management Preparation—Scope of the Problem: "Trust me! I've got this under control!"

In an Australian survey, surgeons asked about particular needs of a crisis training course said the following: [31]

- "The whole persona of a surgeon is somebody who can make quick decisions and cope with anything. Except when things go wrong…. Then that same person can't think straight makes mistakes *and loses all judgment; everything descends into chaos and patient care is seriously compromised because he just crumbles under stress"*

- "Surgery is a stressful environment. Yet the surgical community seldom acknowledges the stress associated with carrying out surgical procedures, possibly because emphasis on leadership and self-confidence is so high that stress is often perceived as a sign of weakness or failure. *There is no systematic institutional strategy for dealing with stress.* Consequentially, inexperienced trainers are not explicitly taught how to manage these intraoperative stressors when they occur and learn to cope only through observing their seniors manage similar scenarios or from making their own mistakes."
- "There is clear evidence that excessive levels of stress have a deleterious effect on performance. As a result high-risk/high reliability industries have introduced stress and crisis-management training to prepare junior trainees to respond effectively and efficiently to on the job stressors."

In this Australian survey on what surgeons desire for training in appropriate mechanisms to react in a crisis, Arora et al, asked surgeons to describe the coping strategies they employed during a crisis. These methods can be broken into four basic categories seen in Figure 19. [31]

When anyone asks a colleague to describe their strategies for perioperative management of intraoperative stress, there is usually a silence followed by some vague descriptors of what they may have seen or thought they did. The Australian survey reflects that surgeons have a minimalistic understanding of the various processes involved in preparation for and surviving as a team during a disaster. As a whole we have some general ideas as to how we prepare and react during these situations, but unlike other high pressured fields, a clear organized process is evidently lacking for surgeons.

PERIOPERATIVE COPING STRATEGIES USED FOR MANAGING AN O.R. CRISIS	
PREOPERATIVE PLANNING AND PREPARATION: • Mental rehearsal of surgery • Briefing with the team • Contingency planning for problems • Checking behavior (patient lists)	**INTRAOPERATIVE COGNITION STRATEGIES:** • Stop, step back and deep breath • Go back a step in the procedure • Self talk • Recall how senior surgeon dealt with it • Remain objective • Verbalized if limitation is reached
INTRAOPERATIVE BEHAVIOR • Minimize distractions • Order more equipment / personnel • Damage Control	**INTRAOPERATIVE TEAMWORK:** • Call for help from seniors • Speak with scrub nurse ("there is a problem! Let's concentrate") • Reassure juniors

Figure 19 Perioperative Coping Processes used for managing an O.R. crisis. You can see that these are very rudimentary, and the diagram does not exhibit that there is a formal organized training process in place. For a complex, dangerous industry, there is a long way to go from this to a more systematic universal protocol on dealing with a crisis.

Arora S, Sevdalis N, Nestel D, Tierney T, Woloshynowych M, Kneebone R. Managing intraoperative stress: what do surgeons want from a crisis training program. *Am J Surg*. 2009;197:537-543. [31]

In the same year, Wiggins reported on a survey of 26 surgical faculty and senior general surgery residents from a single academic health center. Ninety-six percent of the surgeons felt confident and would expect to be successful during a crisis situation. While the majority stated they did not find these situations particularly stressful, 40% did.

Most felt that these skills could be taught, and that practice and preparation were reported as very important. Competence, confidence, composure, preparation, and experience were most commonly listed as characteristics or behaviors that should be encouraged in aspiring surgeons. Anger, panic, indecision, fear, and chaos were the most commonly listed characteristics that should be discouraged. This was however, a self-assessment and there has been no follow-up of these providers to determine their actual temperament and leadership skills during a disaster. [128]

Having said that, Runciman noted the well-known attribute of clinicians, *"optimist bias,"* in which most individual members of a group view and report their abilities as *better than the average*. An additional dangerous phenomenon is the ability of individuals to rely on their more experienced partner's or superior's ability to handle crises from past experience. These individuals are unlikely to be motivated to spend any time or effort on training. [33]

The clinicians, in these cases, did recognize that crises are a challenge for the items noted in Figure 20, below. In addition, this group attempted to explain why some clinicians do not seem to respond appropriately during a crisis. These factors are noted in Figure 21, below. [32-34]

FACTORS PRESENT DURING CRISES WHICH MAKE RESPONSES MORE CHALLENGING		
PRESENCE OF NON-SPECIFIC SIGNS INITIALLY: • Blood pressure change • Pulse Oximetry change • Increase in $ETCO_2$	LACK OF SKILLED ASSISTANCE AVAILABLE DURING THE NECESSARY TIME FRAME	PARTICULAR SET OF CIRCUMSTANCES MAY NEVER HAVE BEEN ENCOUNTERED BEFORE
RECENTLY INTRODUCED VARIABLES BRING ON UNFORSEEN CONSEQUENCES: •Processes •Staff •Equipment	➢INTERACTION OF MULTIPLE COMPLEX ISSUES ➢LAYERS OF COMPLEXITY ADDED AS PROBLEMS ARISE	NEED TO RESOLVE FACTORS FASTER THAN THE TEAM IS CABABLE OF COMPREHENDING WHAT THE SITUATION IS

Figure 20 Factors present during crises which tend to make the crisis more challenging…

Runciman WB, Merry AF. Crises in clinical care: an approach to management. *Qual Saf Health Care*. 2005;14:156-163. [33]

FACTORS RELATING TO INEFFECTIVE PROVIDER RESPONSE DURING A CRISIS		
TRAINED RESPONSE FOR CLINICIANS : ➢SEARCH FOR MORE COMMON PROBLEMS AND SOLUTIONS ➢FOCUS AWAY FROM THE UNUSUAL	RULE-BASED COGNITIVE REASONING TYPICALLY RESULTS IN USING UP APPLICABLE RULES OR APPLYING THE WRONG PRINCIPLE (*)	USE OF KNOWLEDGE-BASED DELIBERATIVE REASONING TYPICALLY ENDS UP SLOWER THAN IS ACCEPTABLE FOR THESE SCENARIOS
CONFIRMATION BIASES AND FIXATION ERRORS ARE RAMPANT	ANXIETY DEGRADES PERFORMANCE	MULTICIPLICITY OF TASKS NEEDED SIMULTANEOUSLY DEGRADES PERFORMANCE

Figure 21 Factors relating to ineffective provider response during a crisis

*Use of pre-stored information and past scenario experience is not necessarily faster if the rules are used up or the wrong ones applied.

Adapted with permission from: Runciman WB, Merry AF. Crises in clinical care: an approach to management. *Qual Saf Health Care.* 2005;14:156-163. [33]

When one takes into consideration the information previously presented on the rarity of these events in any one surgical teams workload, and the fact that current assessment of resident training indicates a marked reduction of O.R. workload and especially complex open procedures, it should be obvious that this sets up most facilities to be in a state of shock when a disastrous event occurs.

History of Crisis Training: "You got a checklist for that?"

Aviators developed a mindset for crisis training and assessment in 1954 when Flanagan introduced the critical incident technique, to reduce the loss of military pilots and aircraft, but it took several disasters in the 1970s to prompt further assessment of the situation and widespread training. [129]

One of the first assessments of the use of military response training in anesthesia was by Cooper in 1978. In the 1950s - 1960s three prior anesthesia groups attempted to look at human error as a cause of anesthesia deaths and reported that between 65% - 87% of deaths were directly caused by human error. Cooper identified, however, that post event assessments were far from helpful in actually assessing all the various causes, similar to the aviation field. [38-41]

Runciman's group of Australian anesthesia providers approached this issue in 1993 after reviewing over 2,000 incidents in the Australian registry. Their group identified that when complex life threatening crises happen the anesthesia team is required to rely upon cognitive tasking above and beyond the information processing capacity of the human brain. They modeled an algorithm approach similar to that used by pilots; they proposed it would cover 99% of emergencies encountered. The initial trial revealed that 1/8 of the anesthesia providers were not able to use the checklist effectively. Their work eventually resulted in a crisis manual; however, their follow-up report in 2005 concluded that **a)** ***experience does not prevent failure,*** and **b)** ***even senior providers make mistakes during crises.*** Their conclusion was that in more than half of the crises, ***the signs were non-specific*** **and** ***did not result in a rapid conclusion in the cause.*** Their examples show that in addition to the trauma to the family and team after the brain death of a thirteen-year old child, the physician in charge of the care of that child was charged with manslaughter due to her failure to recognize an issue with the anesthesia circuit. [32-34]

Regrettably, surgeons overall have not kept pace with our non-medical or anesthesia cohorts on teaching surgeons or surgical teams how to maintain control when the unexpected happens. O.R. disasters can come in many shapes and sizes:

- Disasters *internal* to the O.R. consist of hemorrhage, shock, arrest, major organ injury, anesthesia emergency (airway catastrophe or malignant hyperthermia) and O.R. fires.
- *External* ones could include earthquakes, hospital fire, tornado, an armed patient, bomb threat, or attack, etc. [18]

While aviation teams undergo simulation training to assure that the team can coordinate successful recovery strategies in the face of a crisis, intraoperative surgical crisis management is learned in an unstructured manner if at all. More often this is composed as either individual training (not team training) or simply checklists to manage crises along known pathways based on literature support, but these do not take into consideration the aspects described below.

Moorthy reports on one of the few attempts to measure simulation crisis training. In their study they exposed ten junior and ten senior trainees to a bleeding crisis and measured the trainee's technical ability to control the bleeding and of their teams human factors skills. The results were not surprising: senior trainees scored higher than the juniors for technical skills but there were no differences in human factors skills. This attempt at training does not train an entire team, but simply one individual. [130]

Stages in Team Management at the Initiation of a Crisis, through Deliberation, followed by Risk Management

In this section one will learn to successfully lead their team through navigating the pitfalls of the immediate response to a crisis using adaptive behaviors, practicing effective time critical rapid decision making processes, and following through with successful risk-management strategies. This involves two basic stages.

Stage #1: Immediate Personal/Team Hazard Responses (Adaptive vs. Maladaptive Responses)

Effective team leadership should harbor the ability to control oneself effectively in the crux of a crisis using adaptive behaviors and assist the team in avoiding or recovering from maladaptive behaviors.

In this section we will discuss why we decompensate in the face of stress, and tried and true methods that have enabled others to survive.

Stage #2: Deliberation and Positive Action

This is team control transitioning into time-critical rapid processing of information followed by risk management strategies. In this section we will describe a simple mnemonic for organizing a team for a disaster response then assess the nuances of team leadership, followership, and communication. We will then go into more detail regarding the process of time-critical risk assessment and management strategies.

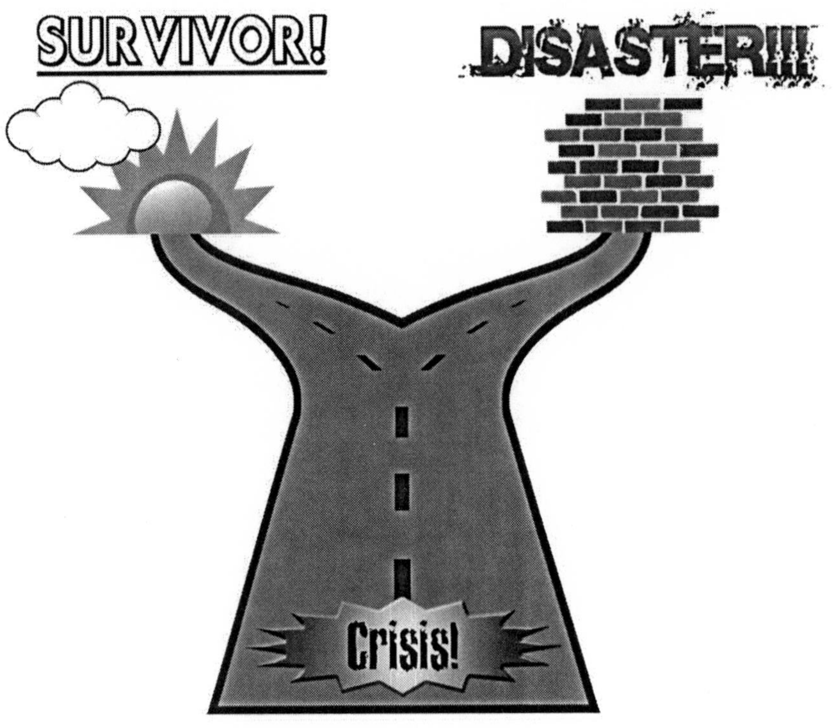

Figure 22 Evolution of an error, accident or other surprise through the stages of crisis evolution with alternative outcomes as an exercise in survival or a disaster.

Adapted from: Seeger, M. W.; Sellnow, T. L., & Ulmer, R. R. Communication, organization and crisis. *Communication Yearbook.* 1998;21: 231–275. [4]

Venette, SJ. *Risk Communication in a High Reliability Organization: PHIS PPQ's Inclusion of Risk in Decision Making.* Ann Arbor, MI: UMI Proquest Information and Learning; 2003. [5]

By this point it should be clear that just because one is a surgeon, trained at dealing with intense risky scenarios, does not mean they will instinctively be capable of steering a team through an unexpected crisis. As a high-risk, high-pressured field, we have a long way to go in the training arena.

There is a pathway to success during a crisis and knowing that in advance is a clear advantage. Figure 23 explores the various phases a team will go through during this process. But before going into the details of the successful response exemplified by survivors, one first needs to explore how surgeons in general perform decision making during task execution in high risk scenarios. The following processes may not occur in the exact same order in all individuals in all circumstances based on the level of preparedness of the individual or team for that particular crisis. Certain overlap of these stages should be relatively obvious, but keen observation of teams in the midst of a crisis would likely yield the majority of these steps in very much the similar order as they appear here.

After a crash course in problem solving in high pressured fields, one needs to understand panic and what causes it. By thinking through these processes one can learn how to succeed in getting through the first few seconds to minutes after a disaster strikes, thereby having the mental capacity to lead the team through to success and recovery. Once the team has a leader and is well-coordinated, risk management and recovery are possible.

Stage 1:
SURVIVAL ARC

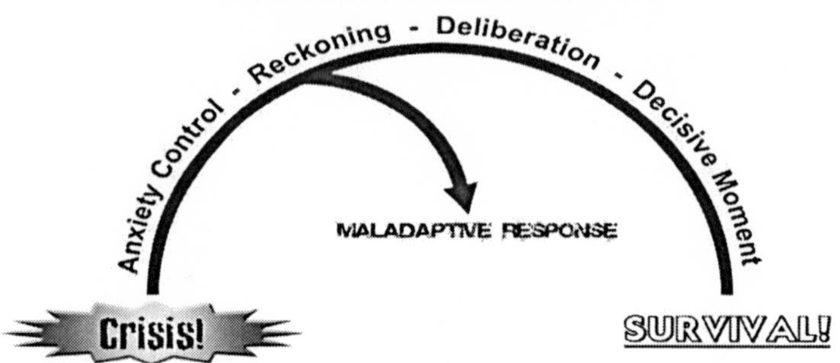

Stage 2:
LEADERSHIP AND COMMUNICATION

Establishment of order via:

- **Team Leadership**
- **Communication**

Stage 3:
DELIBERATE POSITIVE ACTION

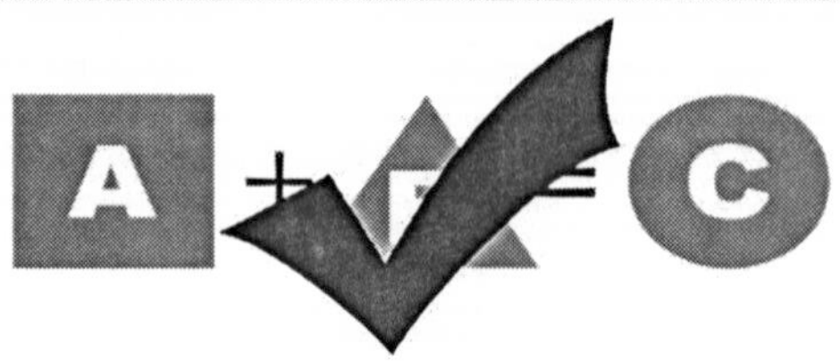

Figure 23 Pathway to Survival! How to overcome the odds in virtually any anxiety provoking situation!
A. **SURVIVAL ARC / COMBAT SURVIVAL TRAINING**: Immediate personal (team) hazard response via adaptive vs maladaptive behavior. Within the first few seconds, individuals must progress through the "survival arc" and either avoid maladaptive behavior or fail. This truly takes Combat Survival Training.
B. **ESTABLISHMENT OF ORDER VIA EFFECTIVE TEAM LEADERSHIP & COMMUNICATION**: Shortly thereafter, the team needs to organize by declaring a leader. Followers must understand who is in charge, their roles and effective communication techniques.
C. **DELIBERATE POSITIVE ACTION PHASE**: Once order has been restored, damage control followed by risk assessment, containment, planning, execution and reassessment are needed.

Problem Solving in Stressful, High Paced Professions: How We Work Through a Problem; "Yes! It Is Important to Understand the Way a Surgeon Thinks and Yes, It Is Logical!"

With the exclusion of time pressures (those that are not typically encountered in surgery), most professionals in high paced careers (i.e. pilots, combatants, first responders, wilderness rescuers, etc.) perform complex decision making in very similar formats.

Figure 24 portrays the normal thought processing that occurs during routine complex cerebral analysis and decision making. As noted previously in Figure 6, page 88, much of the input is processed at a subconscious level and output for routines tends to be subconscious or semiconscious level. Only when we reach the stage at the higher level of Rule-based or into the Knowledge-based processing, do we function at a fully conscious level. When we reach a stage that our mind recognizes there is a problem (hopefully) we wake up and formalize the processing from that point onwards. Keep in mind, however, that all too often heuristics causes confirmation or fixation bias and we function at a lower level than we ought to.

Figure 24 summarizes Pauley's description of problem recognition-solving processes. This can be simplified as follows: [131, 132]

A. The problem is detected.
B. The problem is defined.
C. The overall situation is assessed in four phases:
    1. Threat perception occurs (aspects that pose a threat to the safety of the situation –such as patient underlying condition- anatomy, BMI, adhesions, unexpected findings…)
    2. Risk tolerance assessed (risk surgeon is willing to accept)
    3. Risk assessment (high vs. low)
        - <u>Task complexity</u> – Inaccurate test results, blood loss, laparoscopy issues, etc.

- Environmental—Patient position, broken equipment, etc.
- Other team members—Poor communication, inexperience, bravado, lack of recognition of a problem, etc.
- Organizational—Pressure to keep open conversion rate low, do more cases, acceptance of violation of safety, low resources, etc.

4. Analyze time available (little time vs. more time available)

D. Time Critical—Rapid Process Decision Making Strategies: these occur in four typical methodologies (in order of frequency of use):

1. Analytical (Multiple options weighed and analyzed simultaneously)
2. Intuitive/recognition-primed (RPD) (Familiar event, experience, triggering memories of prior similar events)
3. Rule based (Rules of thumb, documented solutions: i.e, "If 'A' happens, then pack the patient.")
4. Creative (Novel approach)

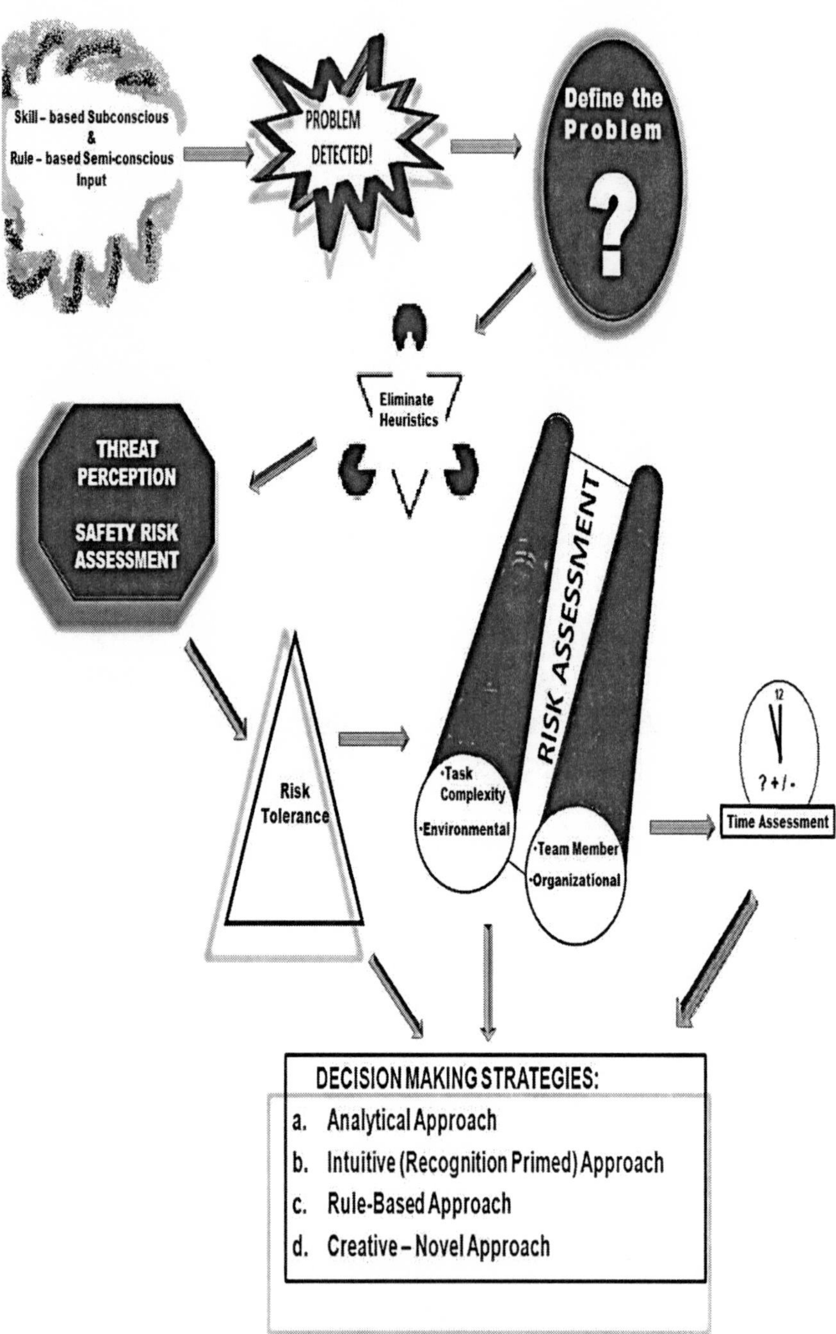
Skill – based Subconscious
&
Rule – based Semi-conscious
Input
PROBLEM
DETECTED!
Define the
Problem
?
Eliminate
Heuristics
THREAT
PERCEPTION
SAFETY RISK
ASSESSMENT
RISK ASSESSMENT
Risk
Tolerance
•Task
Complexity
•Environmental
•Team Member
•Organizational
12
? + / -
Time Assessment
DECISION MAKING STRATEGIES:
a. Analytical Approach
b. Intuitive (Recognition Primed) Approach
c. Rule-Based Approach
d. Creative – Novel Approach

Figure 24 Problem Recognition-Problem Solving Pathways—How we work through a problem: Initially one breaks out of their typical Skill-based subconscious pathway to discover an unexpected problem. Once the problem is detected, the observer must determine what the problem is. If they are successful in eliminating biases and other heuristic errors they must then determine what threat/safety risk the problem poses to their environment. Three processes then must occur: a) determination how much risk the team can tolerate, b) what is the risk to their current objective and team based on what is going on around them, and c) how much time they have. Once that occurs the observer can determine what strategy to use based on one of four common type of problem solving approaches.

Adapted with permission from:

Pauley K, Flin R, Yule S, Youngson G. Surgeons intraoperative decision making and risk management. *Am J Surg*. 2011;202:375-381. [131]

Cohen I. Improving time-critical decision making in life-threatening situations: observations and insights. *Decision Analysis*. 2008;5:100-110. [132]

By this juncture we have reviewed adaptive well-adjusted time critical decision making that occurs in a surgeon typically *not* under tremendous pressure, facing little if any threat. In the average human, when stress and risk are compounded with the unknown, you can typically throw out the organized process noted above and expect anxiety and *panic*!

For anyone to proceed in the systematic manner noted above, they must understand the "fight-or-flight" response, why it happens, what it does, and how you can potentially control this and respond in an organized controlled fashion.

The next section explains our maladaptive fight or flight responses when we have been untrained to control our natural reflexive responses.

Stage #1: Immediate Personal/Team Hazard Responses (Adaptive vs. Maladaptive Responses to a Crisis)

Effective team leadership should harbor the ability to control oneself effectively in the crux of a crisis using adaptive behaviors, and assist the team in avoiding or recovering from maladaptive behaviors.

The first few seconds after a disaster strikes, effective leaders dictate the eventual outcome. Once one understands how surgeons think through stressful circumstances then it is possible to begin to understand advantageous-compensatory-adaptive responses as opposed to disadvantageous- de-compensatory- maladaptive processes which occur when individuals and teams are exposed to a crisis.

These same processes occur in all types of hazardous environments. When faced with a crisis, all individuals in a group traverse what Amanda Ripley describes as the *Survival Arc*. The Survival Arc represents the strategies one uses to recover when horrendous events occur. The Survival Arc occurs in three stages: *Reckoning, Deliberation,* and the *Decisive Moment* (seen in Figure 25).

At each stage, there is a track that leads the participant in the disaster either to success and survival or towards further disaster and potential defeat. The participants must traverse through each stage individually and succeed, to progress to the next phase.

Unfortunately, human nature tends to steer the majority of those exposed to a crisis towards the maladaptive stage rather than towards the goal of success. It would be easy as a bystander observing one of these seemingly inappropriate responses to invalidate the person expressing them. [133]

This is quite frequently seen in hindsight bias where the bystander or reviewer has no idea what the people directly involved were experiencing. In order for one to avoid maladaptive responses in an excessively stressful situation, one must first understand how these arise in the first place.

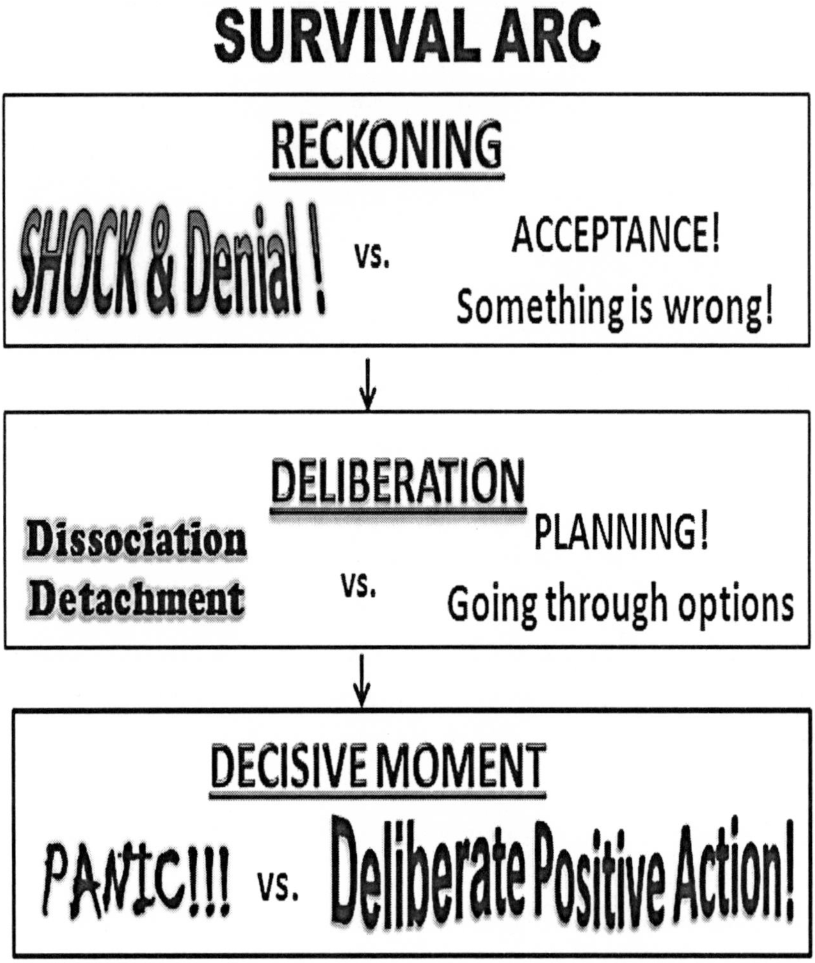

SURVIVAL ARC

RECKONING

SHOCK & Denial ! vs. ACCEPTANCE! Something is wrong!

↓

DELIBERATION

Dissociation Detachment vs. PLANNING! Going through options

↓

DECISIVE MOMENT

PANIC!!! vs. Deliberate Positive Action!

Figure 25 The Survival Arc

Adapted with permission from: Ripley A. *The Unthinkable: Who Survives When Disaster Strikes and Why*. New York, NY: Three Rivers Press; 2009. [133]

Maladaptive Behavior during a Crisis

Origin of Maladaptive Behavior: One of the first questions asked following a crisis or disaster is, "Why did they act like animals?" Why is it during any stressful event, do we behave like we are mindless Neanderthals? Well, in actuality, that is precisely what we are doing. We are acting in an innate, primordial reflexive state.

The simplest explanation can be found in Mathew Sharps' assessment of decision making under stress in law enforcement. Under normal circumstances humans function using the problem solving strategies noted above. Even when something unexpected happens, if this is not threatening and there is time to process the information, this is done at the highest level of human functioning. But, alter the course of events by creating a threat, the need to rapidly process information, and alter one's current course of direction and humans tend to behave a lower level of complexity than expected.

This seemingly paradoxical reflex is exactly that, a reflex. It is an instinct passed along from eons of humans functioning as hunters. When primitive humans were exposed to stress their subcortical functions kicked in as a response of the well-known "fight-or-flight" instinct. This worked well for them as their cortisol and adrenaline kicked in; their trained survival responses were all they needed to win in battle or capture prey. The goal was simply to deliver more oxygen and blood to muscle by diverting it away from unnecessary organs, i.e., the gut and cerebral cortex. They did not need the cortex for these simple actions. Blood was diverted to more effective subcortical areas responsible for their instinctual responses. This resulted in entirely non-discriminatory impulsive behavior based on subcortical performance (see Figure 27, page 169).

This loss of cortical function, especially the frontal cortex, resulted in attention deficit, reduced judgment, a loss of acceptance of alternatives, perseveration, and complete reliance on habitual-instinctive reflexes. This is not bad when trying to run away or to fight a foe or catch a meal, but is maladaptive in the face of a crisis in your operating room.

The same can be said of sympathetically-induced pupillary dilation and loss of lens adaptation during stress. One causes inability to focus at a distance and the other on nearby objects. The loss of depth perception is a low trade-off for the gain in increased light absorption if you are focused on a single target. This can be bad when it creates the potential for blurred vision in the middle of an operative procedure.

Auditory exclusion also occurs under stress where your hearing is entirely focused on the subject that you are facing, to the obliteration of sounds from outside that venue. It is apparent that during stress, when you need more information, your body is shutting your sensory processes down, greatly narrowing your perspective. Again, that is fine if you are focused on your dinner, but not in the middle of a complex procedure that has gone awry.

Tachycardia is an adaptive survivalist response. It appears that optimal response, in times of stress, occurs at heart rates between 115 and 145 beats per minute. In his book on survival motor skills, *Sharpening the Warrior's Edge,* Siddle describes the arousal response on the quality of performance as bell-shaped. Performance for athletes peaks as their arousal enhances up to a point, from which that point forward it begins to deteriorate. One loses fine and complex motor skills starting around 115 beats per minute. Fine motor skills are required by our fingers for operating and complex motor skills are required for integration of hand-eye coordination such as in laparoscopy.

This conundrum poses no problem to the majority of professions that rarely rely on fine motor skill or the hunter chasing his prey or fighting an adversary. Athletes and combatants work well in this range. Unfortunately, this can prove disastrous for the surgeon. To make matters worse, when the heart rate proceeds past 145 beats per minute complex motor function deteriorates. Beyond 175 beats per minute gross motor skills begin to deteriorate—hence an explanation of why people when under stress can be found to freeze, especially when their heart rate jumps to over 220 beats per minute. Figure 26 shows this relationship.

In a stressful situation, an untrained individual recognizes he has encountered something he was not prepared for. This activates an immediate sense of urgency and the need to combat time, thereby escalating the stress even further. The individual's heart rate climbs, quickly paralyzing fine and complex motor skills. Perception disability follows pace, slowing down information processing as well as response programming. A sense of urgency hits the victim, rapidly increasing the heart rate further. The individual now enters the above described fight or flight response.

Trained individuals learn to optimize their *response time* (the time from when they detect a problem till they have completed a task designed to defend them). The total response time is a summation of their *reaction time* (the time that is expended from the moment their sensory system detects a problem, till they respond) and their *movement time* (the time from when they begin the defensive task till it is completed).

Reaction time is generally composed of the length of time it takes your brain to a) perceive a change, b) analyze it properly, c) evaluate it and identify it as a threat, and d) activate a response. Generally speaking, during the course of the majority of surgical procedures this particular training is not of consequence.

Yet, it is that rare episode when something new and unexpected happens that poses a threat, that this response time becomes quite critical. Typically we fail to recognize that something has changed the instant that that change occurred. This is a combination of the heuristic biases noted above, distraction, fatigue, and the fact we are typically hyper-focused.

Unfortunately, this lack of recognition combined with slow response times in an individual due to lack of training, fatigue, or distraction, can mean a substantial difference between either early recovery or failure to recover. This is compounded significantly if the individual is already under stress and susceptible to the negative influences of perceptual narrowing described elsewhere.

It is helpful to train individuals to begin to prepare to be aware by breaking down their response time into these components and analyze their attributes and deficits. You can then focus on your areas of weakness to enhance them. [86-87]

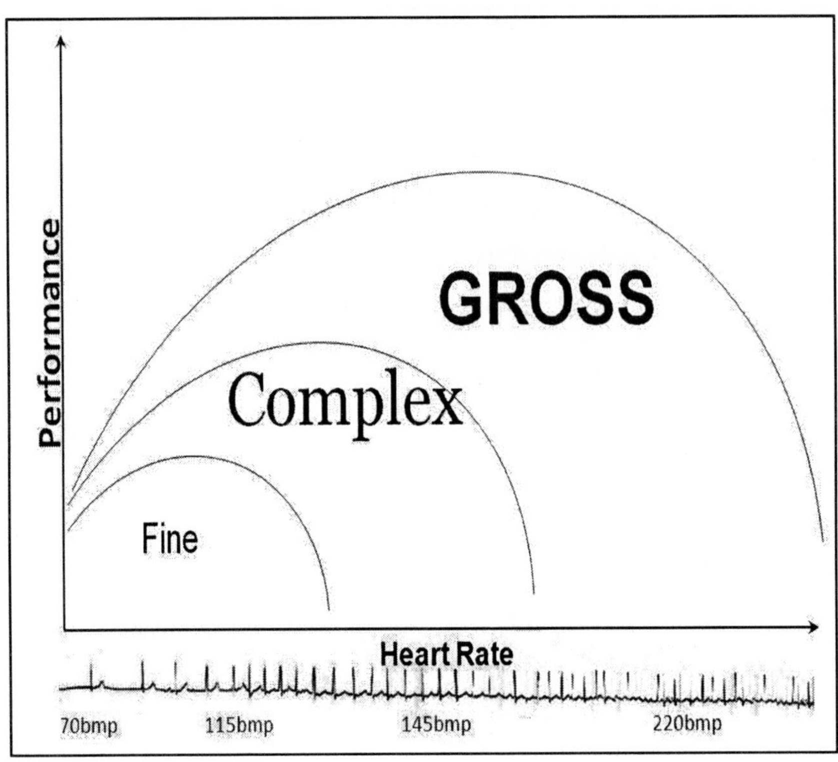

Figure 26 Bell-shaped curve seen when heart rate increases and motor skills are enhanced but then deteriorate.

Adapted with permission from: Siddle B. *Sharpening the Warriors Edge: The Psychology and Science of Training*. 10th ed. Belleville, IL: PPCT Research publications; 2008 [87]

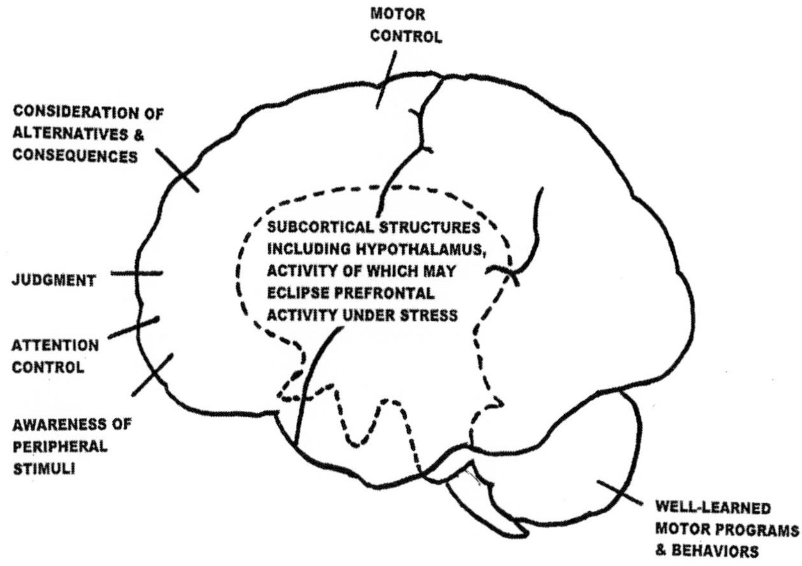

Figure 27 Origins of Maladaptive Responses during Stress
Normal Cortical functions are shut down during stress responses due to the Hypothalamic-Pituitary-Adrenal pathway, resulting in enhancement of the subcortical functions (adversities) noted in the diagram above. [86]

Especially created by Matthew J. Sharps, PhD, DABPS, FACFEI, (Professor of Psychology California State University; Research Consultant, Fresno Police Department), author of *Processing Under Pressure-Stress, Memory and Decision Making in Law Enforcement*, Looseleaf Law Publications, Inc.

Maladaptive Responses to Stress

One of several typical maladaptive scenarios occur in the untrained individual during a crisis encounter (listed in reverse order of potential destructiveness):

1. Sound Anomalies
2. Intrusive Thoughts
3. Automatic Pilot
4. Memory Loss or Distortion of Memory
5. Sense of Time Deceleration
6. Denial
7. Tunnel Vision
8. Dissociation/Paralysis
9. Panic

Here's the breakout:

1. Sound Anomalies: One of the most common responses seen during a crisis, are for sounds to be subjectively diminished in volume (or in some cases louder as the brain selects out specific foci). This can be problematic when one is trying to recover and restore order after a crisis if they cannot focus on voices or important stimuli. [86]
2. Intrusive Thoughts: Mind drift is a common occurrence when one is under pressure. Your prefrontal inhibition allows a multitude of thoughts to enter your subconscious which then interferes with your conscious efforts to resolve the situation. This tendency is exactly what causes loss of impulse

control and lack of diplomacy in some stressful situations. Your random thoughts simply get blurted out. [86]

3. Automatic Pilot: Under stress, many resort unintentionally to habitual, perseverative behavior. They have been trained over and over to respond in a specific way to specific circumstances and even if the situation has changed, their response is unaltered. While typically this is a beneficial response, if the habit is recreated in the wrong scenario, it can be deadly. [86]
4. Memory Loss or Distortion of Memory during a stressful event is a common fact. We get stressed and can't "think straight." We are too rushed to find solutions or a way out. A less commonly known occurrence is losing one's memory of one's actions or events during a crisis. An easy way to prove that is to ask any witness to a crime the details of the events and compare to the recollection of another bystander. The details rarely match. When one is a victim of a crisis, memory loss and distortion is even more profound. [86]
5. Sense of Time Deceleration: Survivors report the sense of time slowing down during a crisis. The perceived sense of speed in the presence of slow-moving surroundings, can lead to a false sense of security. [86]
6. Denial is a heuristic response and is often extremely ironic. This heuristic response is the normalcy-

complacency bias described previously. Recognition of an event as a crisis is a critical process that is frequently overlooked by a team in the midst of a crisis. While on the surface it may seem very basic, participants observing an unfolding disaster first-hand must persuade themselves first and then take on the task of convincing others of the impending doom. Unfortunately, on a basic level, we decide that everything was fine in prior experiences and therefore we must be "okay" in the current but dangerous situation.

Firefighters have often reported coming to a bar or other buildings filled with smoke only to find patrons sitting there drinking and refusing to evacuate. The customers just stated that there was no fire, so there was no reason to be alarmed. Reports of airline passengers sitting in their chairs reading and not realizing a plane engine has blown out and smoking outside their window, is not unheard of. Even when the World Trade Center was under attack, survivors waited an average of six minutes (some more than 45 minutes) before they began to evacuate. In some cases staff were told to "Stay put." Some simply went about making calls or packing belongings. At an average descending rate of one floor a minute and 100 floors to go, occupants did not have that luxury. Normalcy-bias is the situation where we react to past experiences and often this is not a beneficial response. Acceptance that an event is a crisis or disaster is absolutely necessary for a coordinated response, but frequently results in loss of valuable time. [23]

7. Tunnel Vision**:** This is one type of loss of situational awareness. This turns out to be the second most common phenomenon observed during stress. This instinctual response allows the hunter to focus on his prey and ignore invaluable stimuli outside in the periphery. You become focused on what is perceived to be the most important part of the scenario. However, if you become hyper-focused, centrally occupied, valuable information may be lost. It is virtually impossible to lead a team through a crisis if one cannot gather details from the periphery. To make matters worse, this instinctual response is also what is responsible for one ignoring what is obviously in front of them. While this can be hazardous to a surgeon, consider what this response does to one in the military or public protection. Missing a hazard in front, behind, or beside you can then be deadly to you and the rest of your team. [86]
8. Dissociation/Paralysis: This is an extreme example of loss of situational awareness. Dissociation may or may or may not be a positive or disabling response depending on the circumstances. Both of these are more common when individuals experience tachycardia above 170 beats per minute, secondary to cortical flow diversion and dysfunction. *Dissociation* is essentially a detachment from reality. It turns out that Army Special forces candidates who score *high*

on a dissociation screening exam of three questions are *less likely* to make it through the school.

The three basic questions asked are: "Over the past few days have you experienced any of the following: a) things seem to move in slow motion, b) things seemed unreal-dreamlike, or c) you had a feeling of separation from what was happening, as if you were watching a movie?" On the other hand, over one-third of successful soldier graduates of survival school answer, "Yes." Police who successfully survive shootouts tend to act reflexively from training and rely on this dissociation to take over and their automatic impulses to save them. Skill is the ability to do something automatically at the subconscious level without thinking about it. It is programmed by repetition, through practicing over and over until it becomes automatic.

In other professions, dissociation, distraction, and denial can be fatal. After a 1972 Eastern Airline crash into the Everglades, investigators revealed that the pilots were fixated on the landing gear light but unfortunately completely tuned out the warning alarm for their low altitude. After this it was determined that fixation can be fatal and pilots are trained to focus in orderly fashion on their entire instrument panel to avoid dissociation and fixation on the wrong signal. Plus, one person always monitors the altimeter. In many disastrous circumstances, time wasted during dissociation can be the difference between life and death. As explained above, many survivors of the World Trade Center disaster reported seeing others milling around in dissociative activities. [23] Total *paralysis* is much less common but certainly more fatal. It, too, is associated frequently with extreme tachycardia. [86]

9. Panic! Laurence Gonzalez quotes the "four poisons of the mind: *fear, confusion, hesitation, surprise.*" [71] While simplistic in appearance these four mindsets critically disturb the ability to cope with a crisis.

   It essentially takes three conditions required to cause *panic and chaos* Figure 28: [23]

   a. Feeling of being *trapped*
   b. Sensation of *helplessness*
   c. Profound sense of *isolation*

Dread: In addition, there is a component of dread involved. Dread is a result of uncontrollability, unfamiliarity, impossibility, suffering, unfairness, and it is compounded by the degree of destruction.

Control the fear, panic, and chaos! Advice from multiple experts in the area of *shock, denial,* and *delay* on eliminating these from yourself and your team is summarized in the sections that follow.

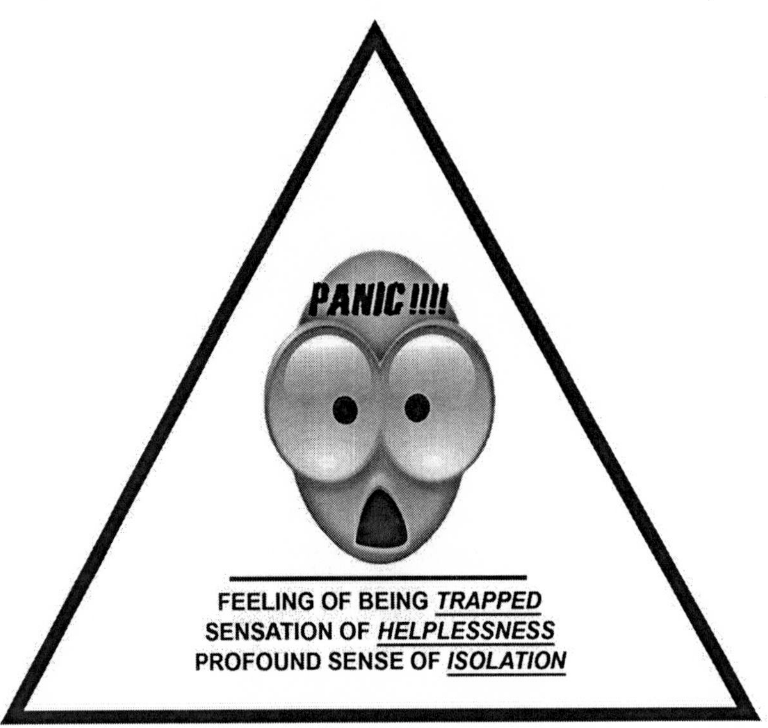

One's tendency to panic is partially based on their *anxiety* levels. There are two levels of anxiety: state anxiety and trait anxiety.

- *State Anxiety* is how we react to a stressful situation
- *Trait Anxiety* is the general tendency to see things as stressful to begin with (resting anxiety level).

Figure 28 Three Conditions are required to cause panic and chaos. These three conditions compounded with dread, typically result in panic. Learning to control these will limit or eliminate panic from a team. Dread is a result of uncontrollability, unfamiliarity, impossibility, suffering, unfairness and compounded by the degree of destruction. [23]

Adapted with permission from: Dörner D; The Logic of Failure: Recognizing and avoiding error in complex situations. Reading MA Perseus Books, 1996. [23]

Those with high trait anxiety are the people who "lose touch with reality when under physical stress" and then overreact. These are the folks who do not tend to survive crises. [23, 134]

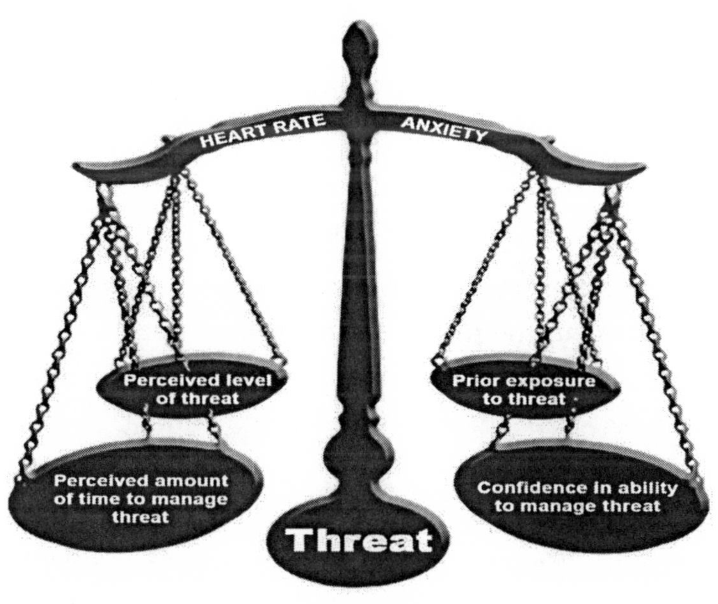

Figure 29 Anxiety is all a matter of balance. Anxiety is all a matter of how you perceive the threat: a) how much of a threat is it to you, b) have you been exposed to this threat before, c) how much time you have to deal with the threat, and d) how much confidence you have in managing the threat. By decreasing anxiety you can decrease your heart rate, gaining control of fine and complex motor function. If any one of these becomes out of balance the threat is perceived as overwhelming, anxiety picks up and the heart rate increases further debilitating the victim.

Adapted with Permission from: Siddle B. *Sharpening the Warriors Edge: The Psychology and Science of Training*. 10th ed. Belleville, IL: PPCT Research publications; 2008. [87]

Combat Survival Training: How Military, First Responder, and Wilderness Rescuers Combat Anxiety in the Midst of Overwhelming Stress and Anxiety

It should be obvious that the faster one moves through the three stages above (reckoning, deliberation, and decisive moment) the higher the chances of survival through any crisis. In terms of the operating room, this can be the difference between survival or death of a patient.

The quicker one is consciously aware of their situation and has completed a situation assessment, the faster they can proceed through these stages. To do this one must train to combat panic. Some of this training begins prior to the crisis.

1. Lower Your Anxiety Level: *Practice to control your fear!*
   - Controlled Breathing: Practice breathing while counting to three, hold for three seconds and exhale while counting to three. This has been a technique taught to military and civilian combatants. It increases your effective lung volume thereby allowing sufficient oxygenation, while at the same time prevents hyperventilation associated with loss of excess CO_2 and its associated cerebral dysfunction. Do this in traffic, waiting in line, at home, and in other stressful environments.
   - Visualization: Just like athletes visualize themselves successfully performing their next move in their mind, trained combatants learn that under stress they can picture in their mind the successful overcoming of the threat in front of them. This in turn primes their body to respond appropriately to the task they face. One successful maneuver is before combatants engage in a risky environment, they mentally prepare for the proper survival response to the most likely adversarial situation they may encounter. They also develop a backup plan and prepare for that as well.
   - Confidence: Perception of Personal Ability to Overcoming the Odds: The survival mindset of a

warrior allows them to face the odds before them in a state where failure is not a focus. The focus is on success. They know they may not survive, but in lieu of focusing on their imminent death, they focus on the threat and environment before them and rely on the tools they have in their possession (including past training). In spite of the possibility of death, they maintain full concentration. This mentality has to do with their confidence, value of life, and belief in the mission. [87] Figure 30 below summarizes multiple techniques used by many survival experts in the face of danger to minimize panic and gain control.

2. Train Your Brain: Prepare for the most likely scenario that you will face. If you are a surgeon, practice in the O.R. with your team! (As an aside, fires kill more people than any other disasters combined; so worry about dying in a fire and train how to respond before worrying about surviving nuclear fallout or another remote event).
3. Be Physically Fit: It is a well-known fact that healthy people survive disaster more often than their unhealthy obese counterparts.
4. Calculate Your Risk: Can you handle it, are you prepared or should you reduce your risk or find someone experienced to help you? Don't go into a procedure or other activity where you are concerned about a high potential for failure without backup.

5. Know Your Neighbors/Coworkers: Your life will *not* be saved by rescue personnel in most instances. This is true in your neighborhood, in the office, and in the O.R. The folks in the room are the ones who will help get the team through the crisis, so the sooner they respect and will follow you through routine high-risk procedures, and will learn effective communications and train with you for an unexpected crisis, the better you will be supported when all hell breaks loose. [70, 71, 133, 135]

FEAR PANIC CHAOS TRAPPED HELPLESS ISOLATED UNCONTROLABILITY UNFAMILARITY IMPOSSIBILITY

URGENCY HELPLESS TRAPPED CHAOS PANIC FEAR

DENIAL DISORIENTATION CONFUSION SURPRISE HESITATION FEAR

- STOP: Maintain calmness by *stopping* what you are doing! Take a break. Repeat to yourself, "Be calm, be silent." Talk the situation through to yourself or others. Use humor. Sing a song or quote a saying to yourself (mantras help eliminate fear in the military during times of stress)! Deep Breathing!
- Think positive! Avoid cataclysmic catastrophic thoughts! Whatever the situation, constantly look for an alternative, a way out.
- Watch for the causes of panic and dread: Trapped, helpless, isolation, uncontrollability, unfamiliarity, impossibility, suffering, unfairness and compounded by the degree of destruction
- Watch for tunnel vision. Stress causes people to focus too narrowly on whatever they thought was most important, but it may be the wrong thing.
- Admit to yourself you are lost, confused and need help!

- Delay and Dissociation is caused by normalcy bias (a type of Confirmation Bias). Recognize the signs you are fixated on "Nothing has changed! All is normal! Everything is okay." We find comfort in the usual.
- Maintain situational awareness. Listen to sights and sounds around. Look for confirmation or contradiction to your sense all is normal—face reality.
- Listen to the voice inside your head. Trust gut feelings.
- Be wary of staying in the skill-based zone (subconscious) for too long, and move to a more conscious rule-based or knowledge-based level of thought.
- If you are observing someone else panicking, help them remove one of the elements so they can move on. For panic and dissociation, get the person's attention by any means possible.

DETERIORATOIN DISORIENTATION FRANTIC TRAPPED HELPLESS ISOLATED UNCONTROLABILITY

Figure 30 Calming the fear, panic, and eliminating dissociation. This summary describes well known techniques utilized by those frequently faced with survival situations to combat panic.

Adapted with permission from:

Gonzales L. *Deep Survival: Who Lives, Who Dies and Why*. New York, NY: WW Norton; 2003. [23]

Ripley A. *The Unthinkable: Who Survives When Disaster Strikes and Why*. New York, NY: Three Rivers Press; 2000. [133]

Survivability: The Survivor's Personality

Finally before moving on to the next steps, one needs to explore the traits of the typical survivor. You need to understand that there is a common pattern to the way survivors handle daily life and life under pressure. You should explore these personality types and explore the various resources available to see how to transform, especially if you clearly do not fit these survival personality characteristics.

A summary on the characteristics of who typically survives a disaster includes:

- Versatile/Tolerate change:
    - During periods of disruptive change, new developments, threats, and confusion they respond by asking, "What is happening?" ** (see key below)
    - Read new situations rapidly. **

- Ability to perceive and believe what is happening around them and adapt to it. **
- Cope during transition. Adapt to new reality. **
- Increased mental and emotional flexibility; Develop many response choices for different situations **
- Know their stuff and have a plan, backup plan and bailout plan, but remain flexible. Are willing to consider any options to recover. **
- Rapidly regain emotional balance. Recover to a stable condition. (Victims attack and blame others.) Do not get trapped by denial. **
- Assume that working with change and ambiguity are a way of life. Handle change with self-confidence. **
- Accept current situation no matter how bad it is. Expect that something can be done to influence events in a positive manner and lead to a good outcome. **

- <u>Organized</u>:
    - Quickly take action by setting up routines, discipline, and manageable tasks.
    - Break large jobs into smaller ones.
    - Have a mantra, such as a military march song.
- <u>Rational but hopeful</u>:
    - Positive mental attitude. Celebrate successes, count their blessings.

   - Avoid cataclysmic thoughts even if odds are against them. Turn any bad situation into an advantage.
- Empathetic: Understand what others are going through.
- Observant: Take time to observe and reflect even during adversity.
- Purposeful: Find a way to be useful in all situations.
- Healthy: Obese, unhealthy people have lower success of surviving threats.
- Calm: Lowered anxiety levels; have control over their anxiety in all situations.
- Not impulsive: Think options through based on information available and consider changes that reflect a change in their environment.
- Humble but self-confident and have a healthy self-concept: the Rambo types are the first to go; those who choose humility can't be reckless or arrogant.
- Help others:
   - Helping others survive is a survival advantage; it takes you above yourself and above your fears.
   - Doctors and Nurses tend to have an advantage because they care for others.
- Self-Reliant: They don't sit and wait for others to bail them out; they make a plan and work it out.
- Resilient: Cultivate resilience characteristics:
   - Believe they can influence what happens to them.
   - Find meaningful purpose through life's turmoil.

- Open minded: Learn from all experiences, both good and bad.

** Key: These levels of performance require one to function at a *knowledge-based* performance level. Survivors are comfortable observing what is going on, consciously and subconsciously, because it is natural to them. They don't accept everything at face value, but consider how that information fits in with what they are observing. They do not simply toss out information that does not make sense at that time but save it for possible use later.

Non-survivors take all this information, place this into a heuristic profile, fit it into a zone of comfort and function back in a *skill-based* level as if nothing has changed.

<table>
<tr><th colspan="2">Survivability: The Survivor's Personality</th></tr>
<tr><td><ul><li>Versatile/Tolerate change</li><li>Organized</li><li>Rational but hopeful</li><li>Empathetic:</li><li>Observant</li><li>Purposeful</li><li>Healthy</li></ul></td><td><ul><li>Calm: Humble but self-confident</li><li>Help others</li><li>Self-Reliant</li><li>Resilient<ul><li>Influence</li><li>Meaningful purpose</li><li>Open minded</li></ul></li></ul></td></tr>
<tr><td colspan="2">Figure 31 Survivability: The Survivor's Personality [71, 133, 136].</td></tr>
</table>

Standard Firefighting Orders

1. Keep informed on fire weather conditions and forecasts.
2. Know what your fire is doing at all times.
3. Base all actions on current and expected behavior of the fire.
4. Identify escape routes and safety zones and make them known.
5. Post lookouts when there is possible danger.
6. Be alert. Keep calm. Think clearly. Act decisively.
7. Maintain prompt communications with your forces, your supervisor, and adjoining forces.
8. Give clear instructions and insure they are understood.
9. Maintain control of your forces at all times.
10. Fight fire aggressively, having provided for safety first.

From *Fire and Aviation Management, Risk Management* at: http://www.fs.fed.us/fire/safety/10_18/10_18.html

Stage #2: Deliberation and Positive Action—Team Control Transitioning into Time-Critical Rapid Processing of Information followed by Risk Management Strategies

S.T.O.P! A Simplified Approach to Survive Any Situation

Once one understands the process to avoid maladaptive behavior, one then needs to explore the steps survivors of a crisis utilized to succeed. We will go through these steps in more detail later, but one has to keep a mnemonic in mind to help them succeed during time of distress.

After constructing a quick and easy outline in mind of how to process all the chaos going on around us during a crisis, we will discuss the various components present during a crisis that must be present to win. Those invaluable components are a) leadership, b) followership, and c) communication. Following these details we will begin an analysis of how to assess risk, formulate plans and manage further risk.

So first, as promised, the simplest algorithm to aid you in guiding any team through any potential disaster has been described by Laurence Gonzales, as: ***S.T.O.P. or Stop!, Think!, Observe!, Plan!*** This mantra has proven itself in virtually any crisis situation whether it is in the wilderness, open sea, hostage situation, fire, earthquake, career disasters, Operating Room, etc. The primordial step to avoid panic and confusion in the first few moments during a crisis and the most successful pathway to survival is the mnemonic ***S.T.O.P*** (found in Figure 32). [71, 134, 137, 138] We will cover more details about decision making and risk management during a crisis, but this is the best first step.

S.T.O.P. means:

1. **SIT**: STOP everything! Follow the advice in the above section to control anxiety, fear, panic and dissociation.
2. **THINK**: Get organized. Set up manageable tasks. Don't think of the impending goal, only of the next immediate step. Getting out of the room before you are late to the office is *not* the next step. Forget all your other obligations.
3. **OBSERVE**: Perceive and believe. Remember that denial is counterbalanced by recognition, acknowledgement, and acceptance of their situation.
4. **PLAN**: Be bold but cautious while carrying out tasks.
5. **ACT**: Surprisingly, according to several aviation and military experts interviewed, one of the most common mistakes omitted by a distressed person is the need to *act*; that is, they frequently simply forget, or are afraid to move forward with a plan and begin to plan the next step.

On the surface this may appear too simplistic and the further details will be covered later, but one must remember that when you are stressed and full of adrenaline, until you have personally recovered and avoided maladaptive responses, this may be the only method you can remember! [71, 134, 137, 138]

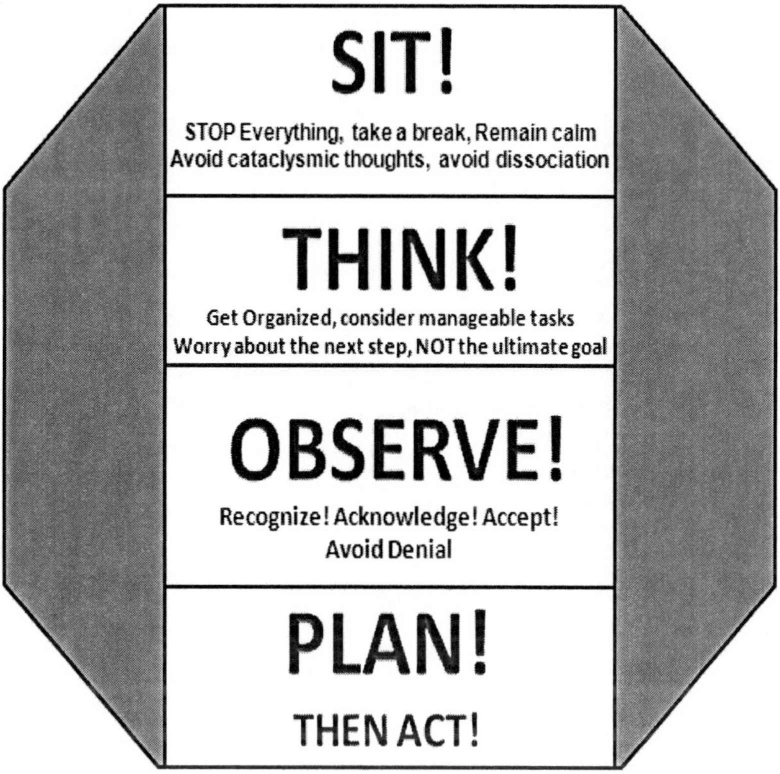

SIT!

STOP Everything, take a break, Remain calm
Avoid cataclysmic thoughts, avoid dissociation

THINK!

Get Organized, consider manageable tasks
Worry about the next step, NOT the ultimate goal

OBSERVE!

Recognize! Acknowledge! Accept!
Avoid Denial

PLAN!

THEN ACT!

Figure 32 Pathway to success in surviving a disaster [71, 134, 137, 138]

Getting Lost: How Did We Ever Get So Lost?

One of the important aspects of controlling surprise, panic, etc. in the O.R. is to understand how we got "lost" in the first place. Remember that running into trouble in the Operating Room is often quite the same as getting lost. We start off with one plan in mind and stick to it even when the environment is changing and we don't recognize it. It is easy to get lost if you do not update your mental map of what is going on around you and instead persist in going the same direction even if the landscape tells you, you are not where you are supposed to be.
<u>Stages of being lost</u>: 1. Denial of disorientation and pressing on. 2. Realization you are lost. Urgency presses in. Thoughts and actions become frantic and unproductive. 3. Expend energy in finding the place that fits your mental map. 4. Deteriorate mentally and emotionally. 5. Resignation to plight, reorient map, develop new plan or die.
Figure 33 Getting Lost Adapted with permission from: Gonzales L. *Deep Survival: Who Lives, Who Dies and Why*. New York, NY: WW Norton; 2003. [23] Ripley A. *The Unthinkable: Who Survives When Disaster Strikes and Why*. New York, NY: Three Rivers Press; 2000. [133]

Leadership: Team Command, Team Dynamics, and Risk Management: "Hey! Somebody's Gotta Take Charge Here!"

Once the individual or team has managed to control chaos and panic, the next steps for the team in surviving the disaster surround leadership and assessment as follows:

Leadership—Commander

Someone needs to take command, take charge. It is important for someone to take control over the situation.

In the majority of organizations, leadership during a crisis is virtually pre-established due to staff hierarchy—that is, the higher ranked or more senior person assumes leadership. That is not quite true in the current medical environment where there exist two if not three independent levels of leadership within the surgical theater: the surgeon and his assistants, the anesthesia team, and the nursing team. For this reason, realms of leadership must be clear to avoid confusion and anarchy.

WARNING! REMEMBER!

1. *The noose always feels much tighter when it's around your own neck!* If the crisis was created by your own error, give a lot of thought whether you should be commanding. Think very hard about turning over

the command to another experienced person if you sense your judgment is clouded by your own anxiety.

2. The Commander cannot be preoccupied with every detail or very specific aspects of the event or he will be unable to maintain total control over the situation.

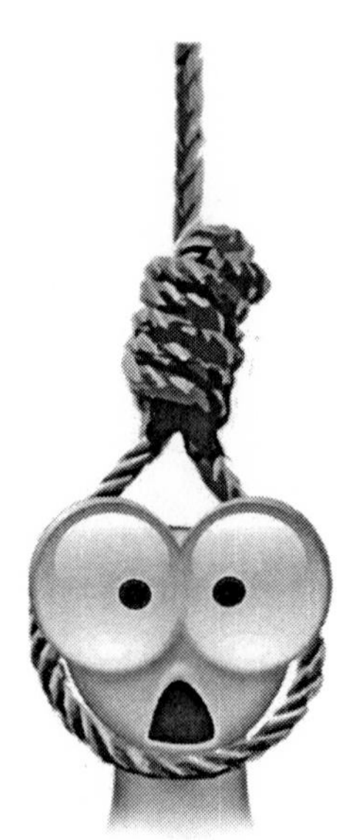

Figure 34 The noose is always tighter when it is around your own neck. Use good judgment when deciding to remain as commander. Reconsider if your judgment may be clouded by anxiety, secondary to a misadventure created by your own error.

Warning! *The person most qualified to lead through a crisis may not be the most senior member of the team, especially when considering the issues brought up above.*

Leadership = Commanding Authority

1. Authority with Respect is maintained by assertiveness over the team using the Coast Guard CRM principle of "authority with participation, yet assertiveness with respect." It is invaluable to remain courteous and considerate of others in the midst of a crisis. Discounting other's importance through disregard, criticism, and screaming only amplifies existing stress.
2. Respectful Clear Communication is not a vain-humble authority but one of assertiveness with complete, directed communication of ideas, wants and needs. This begins with a clear statement to get everyone's attention.
3. Inclusive of Crew-Team input: Concerns must be expressed as "owned emotions," that is, everyone has a personal part in the outcome of the situation. Your statement of the situation must acknowledge if the problem is real or perceived. A quick solution needs to be offered followed by consensus or concise discussion of realistic alternatives. This immediate communication needs to succinct and clear, i.e. just "say what needs to be said." [139, 112, 113]

Commander's Roles

As seen in Figure 35, page 200, the Commander must fully comprehend his/her roles which include, but are not limited to:

1. Develop and lead *The Plan* to overcome the crisis, while processing under pressure (using techniques described below under "risk management").
2. Practice authority with respect.
3. Be respectful.
4. Use clear communication (see below).
5. Be inclusive of Team input.
6. Establish and prioritize tasks with clearly defined goals.
7. Assign roles and workload distribution evenly and appropriately, yet avoid over-tasking individuals, and simultaneously assure the task to appropriate skill levels. Beware of the "I can do anything" attitude in some members. Studies in the 1990s by Dr. Robert Helmreich concluded that commercial airline pilots believe they are immune to work overload.
   Pilot training during that time period included the indoctrination that they "can do anything." Under stress, pilot performance was not as good as they perceived and many failed to recognize they were overloaded and making mistakes.
8. Manage Resources: Declare emergency early and call for help early; key players should not be leaving the room.

9. Recognize and manage conflict resolution, team stress and panic using effective listening, avoiding emotions, remaining focused.
10. Control "Followership." (See Figure 36, page 201.)
    - Assure that "Followership" skills are optimized. The leader and followers must remember that a team is composed of a leader who gives clear directions and followers who are able to think and follow directions.
    - Followers should maintain:
        - Respect for authority.
        - Establishment of Assertiveness/Authority balance—Challenging authority with proper decorum when there are safety concerns.
        - Personal Safety.
        - Safety of Fellow Followers and leaders.
        - Acceptance that authority goes with responsibility.
        - Knowledge of the limits of your own authority.
        - The desire to make the leader succeed.
        - Possession of good communication skills.
        - Development of positive learning attitude.
        - Ego balance and check.
        - Communication to assure the team has clear assignments.
        - Acceptance of direction and information as needed.
        - Reporting of any personal mistakes (This is *not* the time to hide one's errors).

- Constant reports of work.
- Flexibility.

- Control non-productive hazardous emotions:
    - Anti-authoritarian: "Don't tell me what to do!"
    - Impulsivity: "We gotta do something *now!*"
    - Invulnerability: "It can't happen to me."
    - Machismo: "I can do anything and survive."
    - Resignation: "I give, whatever you say…"
    - Pressing: "Come on guys, let's get done with this, we gotta go."
    - "Air Show": "We've always done this; it's fine."

11. Assure the team maintains Situational Awareness through perpetual vigilance. In the midst of a crisis, situational awareness has three components (See Figure 37, page 202):
    - Awareness
    - Reality
    - Perception

    Situational awareness is lost in crises in many professions due to:
    - Ambiguity: more than one interpretation of the situation is possible.
    - Distraction: attention is being diverted from the original point of focus.
    - Fixation: (see below).
    - Overload: too much is happening at one time.

- Complacency: false sense of comfort, masking impending further danger (not out of the woods yet)
- Improper procedure: Deviation from SOP's w/o justification
- Unresolved discrepancy: conflicts in communication, visual input, or conflicting conditions
- Lack of leadership: No one is flying the plane. (see also http://www.montgomerycountymd.gov/content/firerescue/safetychief/ppt/ssd/MCFRS CollisionSafetyStandDownCRMintheCab.pps)

12. Remain cognizant of, and manage errors: Minimization of further errors is a key role of leadership and crew during a disaster. This occurs through:
    - Maintaining situational awareness (see above).
    - Following *tried and true* standard SOPs and Crisis Checklists. This takes the guesswork out of many steps and eliminates arguing over protocols. Pilots who ignored an SOP are 1.6 times more likely to commit a second error.
    - Minimize distractions.
    - Ask before all actions if that step makes sense.
    - Fixation errors are most common but be wary as well of Causation/Over-steering; the hands follow the eyes phenomenon; and Complacency-Risk Taking.

Common Fixation Errors that Occur during a Crisis

1. "One goal-one solution" error (the misbelief that "There has to be only one problem.")
2. Exclusion error ("It has to be anything but this.")
3. Denial ("Everything is fine.")

I AM TEAM COMMANDER HERE!

- Develop, Activate and Monitor ***THE PLAN*** to get us out of trouble!
- Declare an emergency early on!
- Maintain authority with respect!
- Communicate in a respectful, clear manner AND maintain that communication basis throughout the entire team!
- Be inclusive of team input!
- Manage resources effectively!
- Establish and prioritize tasks with clearly defined goals!
- Assign role-workload distribution evenly and appropriately to capabilities!
- Recognize non-productive behavior, such as team conflict, non-productive emotion, stress and panic!
- Control non-productive behavior using effective listening, avoiding personal emotions, remaining focused!
- Maintain team situational awareness!
- Remain cognizant of fixation errors!

Figure 35 Team Command and Controlled Risk Management [7, 112, 113, 139]

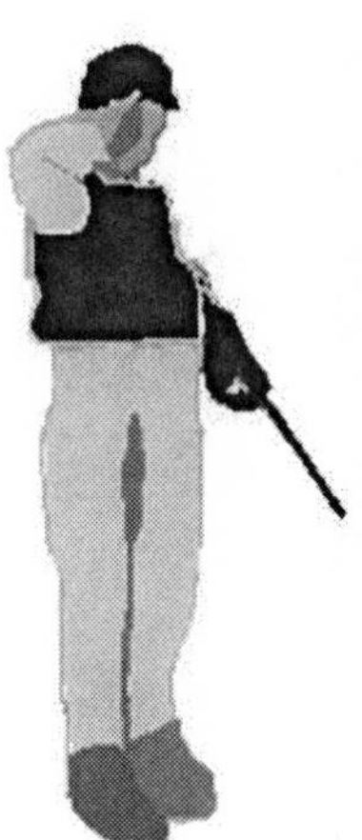

AS A "FOLLOWER" I RESOLVE TO MAINTAIN:

- Respect for authority
- Establishment of assertiveness / authority balance
- Personal safety
- Safety of fellow followers and leaders
- Acceptance that authority goes with responsibility
- Knowledge of the limits of your own authority
- The desire to make the leader succeed
- Possession of good communication skills
- Development of positive learning attitude
- Ego balance and check
- Communication to assure I have clear assignments
- Acceptance of direction and information as needed
- Reporting of any personal mistakes
- Constant reports of work
- Flexibility

Figure 36 Followerism [7, 112, 113, 139]

Components of Situational Awareness

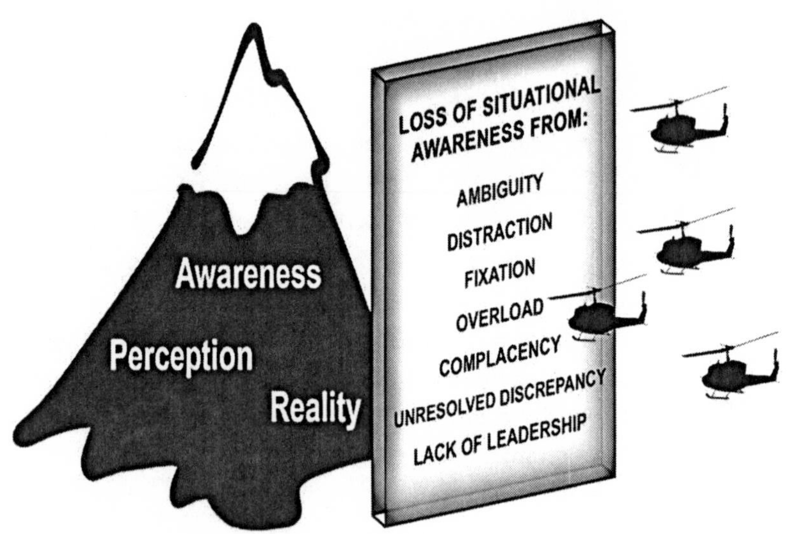

Figure 37 Situational awareness [81, 112, 113]

Team Leadership Skills: Good or Bad "Mayor"?

Surgeons need to be capable of performing a self-assessment to see if they have the leadership abilities to lead the team to success as opposed to the team following the surgeon over the cliff.

Dörner describes the science of successful leadership during a crisis in his book *Logic of Failure: Recognizing and Avoiding Error in Complex Situations.* In his book, Dörner described a study whereby test subjects participated as "mayor" of a fictitious town of Greenville. Greenville was designed to be a complex system of interlocking, ecological, and political components.

Two distinct personalities came out of the experiment: the Successful/ Good Mayor and the Unsuccessful/Bad Mayor, seen in Figure 38. Understanding these characteristics is key to any potential leader in leading any team through success in any disaster. [23]

Good and Bad "Mayor"

SUCCESSFUL / GOOD "Mayor"	**UNSUCCESFUL / BAD "Mayor "**
Innovative and stable.	Unstable.
Made more good decisions than bad.	Focused on less important but more easily solved issues.
Made more possibilities for influencing the fate of Greenvale.	Took events at face value and regarded them as unconnected.
Considered not just the primary goal but also its potential effects on other sectors of the system.	Changed the subject under discussion far more, when they encountered a difficult situation.
Acted more complexly: decisions took different aspects of the entire system into account, not just one.	Exhibited ad-hocism; they are too ready to be distracted.

Asked more *why* questions, about causal links behind events.	Aimless switching of fields of focus at one point and single mindedness; preoccupation with a project to the exclusion of all else.
Able to reach a decision that is totally different than a prior decision.	Decisions always resemble prior decisions.
Find ways to focus on the right fields of endeavor and continue to focus on those fields over time.	Merely recapitulate their behavior.
Reflected on own behavior, made efforts to modify behavior.	Walks away from difficult problems or solves them by delegation.
Capacity to tolerate uncertainty	No capacity for uncertainty

Figure 38 Characteristics of a Good vs. Bad "Mayor" in the Greenville experiment.

Adapted with permission from: Dörner D. *The Logic of Failure: Recognizing and Avoiding Error in Complex Situations.* Reading, MA: Perseus Books; 1996. [23]

Communication

Communication problems were identified as a key component in the majority of adverse events in multiple studies indicated above. This is even truer during a crisis where communication must be accurate, succinct, and in a manner that is accepted by the recipient. Failure of communication will hinder successful progress through the situation.

In the site of the crisis, Communication must remain *accurate*:

- Controlled: voices should remain calm, steady, loud enough to be heard but without shouting.
- Commands need to be accurate, bold, clear, concise, and precise.
- Addressed to specific staff, not global commands.
- Close looped communication—needing constant feedback. Ask, "Does everyone understand me?" Open-ended questions function even better. Ask, "What did you understand I said?" or "What did you hear me say?"
- Open, inclusive exchange.
- Focused on what is right and not who is right

In the site of the crisis, Communication must not be *erroneous* (see Figure 39 for quick summary). Examples:

- Sender:
    - Not establishing a frame of reference: receiver is not on the same page as you.
    - Omitting information.
    - Providing biased-weighted information.
    - Forgetting that body language is important.
    - Forgetting to repeat—We normally talk about 125 words a minute and think at 500-1000 words a minute.
    - Giving disrespectful communication.

- Receiver:
    - Listening with bias, preconceived notions.
    - Poorly prepared to receive information, not consciously ready.
    - Thinking ahead of the sender, extrapolating the information, finishing sentences.
    - Missing non-verbal signals.
    - Not requiring clarification.
    - Disrespectful.

Unfortunately selective filters frequently occur during transition of information from the sender to the recipient's cognitive processing. These filters can easily distort the information resulting in misleading or erroneous interpretations, quickly resulting in inappropriate or dangerous actions on behalf of the recipient.

Filters to be aware of:

- Confirmation bias-resistance to change opinion, even when there is no support.
- Defensive stature.
- Blaming others.
- Halo effect: the infallible one must be right, or "I am right; I am the infallible one."
- "Odd man out" – "I just don't fit in." or "He does not fit in."
- Fatigue.
- Complacency.
- Recklessness.

Other communication issues to be aware of:

- Inquiry: Are you asking the right question, in the right manner of the right person?
- Advocacy: Are you an advocate of your team, mission, and position?
- Listening: Were you really listening? Did he really hear me?
- Conflict resolution: What is right, not who is right.
- Feedback: to confirm understanding.

ACCURATE COMMUNICATION:

- Controlled! Steady! Calm!
- Accurate! Bold! Clear! Concise! Precise!
- Addressed to specific staff- NO GLOBAL COMMANDS
- Closed loop communication with feedback
- Open inclusive exchange
- Focus on WHAT is right and NOT WHO is right!

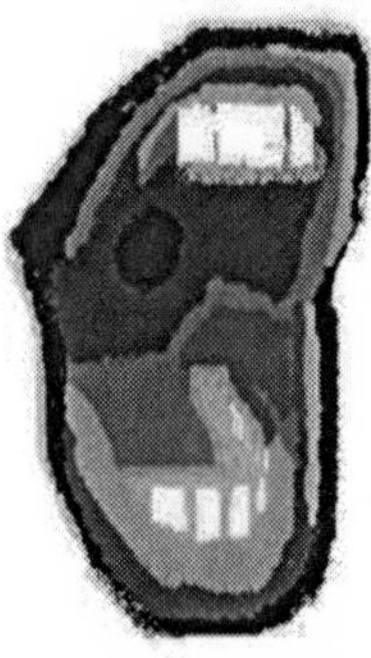

FILTERS

- CONFIRMATION BIAS
- DEFENSIVE STATURE
- BLAMING OTHERS
- HALO EFFECT
- "ODD MAN OUT"
- FATIGUE
- COMPLACENCY
- RECKLESSNESS

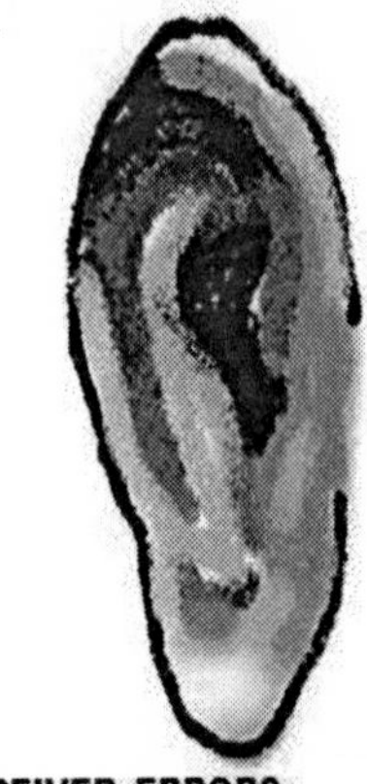

SENDER ERRORS:

- Not establishing a frame of reference
- Omission
- Biased-weighted information transmitted
- Forgetting body language is important
- Forgetting to repeat
- Disrespectful

RECEIVER ERRORS:

- Biased-preconceived notions
- Not consciously ready
- Thinking ahead of the sender
- Extrapolating the information based on biases
- Missing non-verbal signals
- Not asking for clarification
- Disrespectful

Figure 39 Key aspects of communication errors during crisis and selective filters during interpretation [7, 112, 113, 139]

Processing under Pressure: Time Critical Damage Control; Risk Assessment, Management Containment, and Reassessment

As noted above, if all you can remember is the S.T.O.P mnemonic during a disaster, then that will prompt other memories on how to manage the situation. The details surrounding preliminary problem solving thought processes, containment of panic, establishment of leadership and communication rules in crises encountered by high paced professional teams, were discussed in preceding sections.

Once these steps are rapidly commanded, the team needs to move towards the analysis, planning, action, and reassessment stages. This is predominately the role of the team leader, the commander. It is his or her job to move the team past the early checkpoints (noted above) surrounding early containment of the crisis and move the team forward through the decision making processes while under tremendous pressure, often with minimal information, minimal resources immediately available and as rapidly as possible.

Various fields have a multitude of methodologies (and mnemonics) to describe this process, some simplified and some extremely complex.

Quick Summary of Time Critical, Rapid Decision Making Steps Required While under Pressure

These steps should be committed to memory so you can break things down when under fire.

In *Logic of Failure,* Dörner describes Five Simple Steps to *successfully lead through a Complex Situation Crisis.* [23] These five simple steps are:

1. Define your goals: Stay simple and begin with very simple steps. Do not attempt to be too complex. It is not always immediately obvious what you want to achieve
2. Develop a model and gather information: In a crisis, the gathering of information may be limited but it is extremely vital to avoid failure.
3. Prognosis/prediction and extrapolate: Use information gathered to determine potential for success of goals. What can we expect the outcome to be? Should we follow established practice or strike out in new direction?
4. Planning of actions and *execution*: Use simplest possible steps to obtain goals and be alert for biases.
5. Reassessment and Revision of Strategy: Review effects and revision of strategy planning.

FIVE STEPS TO SUCCESSFULLY LEAD THROUGH A COMPLEX SITUATION CRISIS:

1. Define your goals.
2. Develop a model and gather information.
3. Prognosis/prediction and extrapolate.
4. Planning of actions and *execution.*
5. Reassessment and Revision of Strategy.

Figure 40 Five Goals for successfully navigating a crisis.
Adapted with permission from: Dörner D. *The Logic of Failure: Recognizing and Avoiding Error in Complex Situations.* Reading, MA: Perseus Books; 1996. [23]

Prognosis/Prediction: Risk Management Assessment

Prognosis/prediction is known as Risk Management Assessment which involves:

1. Sizing up the probability of successful or poor outcomes.
2. Assessment of the severity of failure.
3. Risk exposure to team, equipment, others in the vicinity (patient).
4. Risk to the mission.

There are many acronyms used by multiple high pressure occupations facing crises situations as a part of their daily activity. Here are a few examples:

- U.S. Fire Administration: The Fire Administration uses one of the simpler formats. They have a modified version of the *D.E.C.I.D.E.* protocol, originally developed in 1978 by NTSB Hazardous materials Specialist, Ludwig Benner.

D Determine the problem.
E Evaluate the scope of the problem
C Consider available options for mitigating the problem.
I Identify the most appropriate option.
D Do the most appropriate option.
E Evaluate the effectiveness of actions.

The original Benner protocol was:

Detecting HM presence,
Estimating likely harm without intervention,
Choosing response objectives,
Identifying action options,
Doing the best option,
Evaluating progress

International Association of Fire Chiefs
Emergency Response Algorithm

D	Determine the problem.
E	Evaluate the scope of the problem.
C	Consider options for mitigating problem.
I	Identify the most appropriate action.
D	Do the most appropriate action.
E	Evaluate effectiveness of actions.

Figure 41 International Firefighters Emergency Response algorithm modeled after Ludwig Benner's Hazmat Emergency Response training model. [140, 141]

- US COAST GUARD RISK MANAGEMENT SCHEME: In the Coast Guard the risk management scheme is much more complicated. In this scheme, the "potential risks to the aircraft and crew shall be weighted against risks to the personnel and/or property in distress if the mission is not taken." "Probable loss of an aircrew is not an acceptable risk."

USCG RISK ASSESSMENT PATHWAY		
STEP #1: PEACE Identify hazards and risk factors: ➢Planning ➢Event complexity ➢Asset selection ➢Communications ➢Environmental conditions	**STEP #2: SPE** (Risk assessment model) Risk = Severity x Probability x Exposure ➢Severity = potential consequences measured in terms of degree of damage, injury or impact on a mission. DAMAGE CAN INCLUDE: Injury or death, equipment damage, mission degradation, morale reduction, adverse publicity, administrative / disciplinary actions	**STEP #3: STARR** Options in management ➢Spread out ➢Transfer ➢Avoid ➢Accept ➢Reduce
STEP #4: EVALUATE RISK vs. GAIN Reality Check! ➢Analyze the operation's degree of risk with proposed controls in place ➢Determine if operational benefits exceed the degree of risk the operation presents ➢Consider cumulative risks	**STEP #5: EXECUTE** ➢The risk control decision is made ➢Clear communication of decision clarifies rationale behind risk management decision	**STEP #6: MONITOR** ➢Monitor situation to ensure controls are effective and in place ➢Identify any and all changes requiring further risk management and act on them ➢Risk management is a continuous process

Figure 42 Risk Assessment Pathway Utilized in Coast Guard CRM Crisis training
http://www.uscg.mil/hq/cg1/cg113/cg1131/riskmanagementpage.asp

If one now returns to the previously described coping strategies utilized by surgeons, in Arora's Australian review on training *Surgeons to React in a Crisis*, (Figure 19), you can see that the field of surgery has not put nearly the amount of thought into how we should be appropriately training surgical teams to respond to a crisis. It should be obvious that various other high pressured field applications should be taken into account.

Team Leadership While Processing under Pressure—A More Detailed Analysis

There are two general speeds of processing during a crisis. Which one works best for you depends on your level of authority and how close to the front you are.

Combat or tactical mode is fast, innate, instinctive, and extremely focused towards a specific target. In this mode you are not paying attention to details.

Detail analysis or strategic mode is slow, focused on the details, mostly observant and interrogatory. In this mode, you observe the situation at hand, take in information from various sources, formulate a plan based on prognostication of success or failure, enact the plan, then reassess and regroup.

Combat mode works very efficiently when you have a mission, are dropped into a specific assigned location, have all the facts up front regarding expected terrain and foe ahead, *and* you have been provided all the skills you need to be prepared long before the mission was engaged. To get there required intense training in the *detailed analysis mode,* to be certain you knew every aspect of your role and what you were about to face. This required repetitive actions until the mission was successful 100% of the time. We learn surgery step-by-step, instrument-by-instrument, until we know the anatomy and effects of each of our actions on the patient.

Combat mode does not work well for a commander who has just encountered an unexpected event requiring time critical rapid decision processing under pressure with little or no information to make a rational decision. Frequently novices dive straight into a crisis with a Rambo mentality only to be in-over-their-heads faster than they can recover. Commanders must learn to control their emotions and hypothalamic-pituitary-adrenal fight or flight response quickly then begin a controlled critical analysis of the situation before things begin to really heat up. This is not an innate behavior, but one the majority of us must learn then practice repetitively until it is natural, innate. Unfortunately it is human nature to quickly look at a situation, see a couple of options, then base a decision on whatever seems to be the quickest way out. This can be seen under the prior section titled "Time Critical Rapid Process Decision Making Strategies" above. The typical response is to choose something we have seen or learned before without a second thought as to whether this is really the best option or consider there may even be other options.

The analytical approach of looking at various options carefully is seldom used by anyone especially when faced with a crisis. We simply do not naturally think in that manner. In a static environment that typically works just fine, but in the midst of a crisis where we have an unexpected change in the environment, with a need to make decisions rapidly, and the mission is threatened, picking the quickest way out without considering other options is not a safe bet.

Taking the time to analyze a situation, consider options and choosing the better option should not be confused with indecision and dawdling (the old "fish or cut bait" dilemma). This process should not be expected to take a considerable amount of time. One just has to make sure they avoid a knee-jerk reflex and truly do an assessment before leading their team towards failure just because they were too anxious and failed to calm themselves and their team.

You may be asking, "How do we change this behavior?" The answer is to be educated first on how effective commanders make critical decisions effectively. They do this in several steps. The first step is learning to train themselves and their team to obtain/provide information that is:

- Accurate and relevant to the situation.
- Provided in a manner that is amenable to your understanding the information so you can then interpret it.

To successfully obtain information with these two qualities, you must be certain the team knows they must provide that information in an *explicit* and *non-inferential* context. They must be trained either in advance or by you telling this up front, that the information must be provided so that all the important elements are connected explicitly. That is, it has to be clear; either they are tied together or they are not tied together. If the provider of information (or you as the commander) infers that information is related without specifically stating so, you (or your team) will not know why something happened or what exactly happened or how it all relates to other events. You may then find yourself sorting through events, binding wrong ones together, and wasting valuable time on the wrong facts. In essence, your decisions must be preempted with all the appropriate knowledge up-front.

This is the concept Mathew Sharps refers to as "front-loaded" information. As commander, you are obligated to do the same thing. You must tell the team exactly what just happened, or why you want them to do what you just requested them to do. You can never assume they will simply "get it." If one now goes back to the original section on human cognitive error, you can see that compiling information left to inference lends itself to fixation errors and then jumping to conclusions. [86]

What type of information exchange are you looking for in a crisis? *Front-loaded and very explicit!*

The next process that a commander and his team have to understand is how human memory works. To assume that you or your team will be able to comprehend a dozen different orders or facts without tying it together in bundles is doomed to failure. In general, as noted previously, humans typically can tackle three to four bundles of information simultaneously. The maximum amount we can integrate is approximately seven organized bundles of information. Having said this, in desperate situations, pulling out the white boards may be your best bet to assure all the information is being distributed and assimilated properly. Remember never to assume!

What really happens when under pressure? Typically when thing go wrong:

1. You first believe you have everything under control.
2. You probably do not alert the team that something has gone dreadfully wrong.
3. You are confident at first that you can rely on your training (or maybe a more experienced partner) and experience to succeed (over confidence).
4. Shrugging off a sense of panic, you push forward (you did not stop to control your heart rate, and now you are in combat mode).
5. The patient continues to bleed from multiple areas by this point.
6. You become focused on the disaster that was created for some time, as the condition begins to deteriorate

(you have now missed the "call an emergency early" mark).

7. You rapidly develop tunnel vision and miss what is going on in the periphery.
8. You may "ignore" questions and details from around you because in reality, you don't hear them (Maladaptive loss of hearing) and have determined you know what is going on anyway (jumping to conclusions- and fixation errors).
9. You consider that you have taken care of hundreds of trauma cases so this should be no different but forget that a) this was totally unexpected, b) you may have created the situation yourself, and c) there may have been other events you were not aware of.
10. You suddenly become aware of what is going on around you and hear bits and pieces of information.
11. Mentally you tie all this information into a scenario that you can handle and begin to bark orders to those in the room (missed the opportunity to obtain explicit front loaded information and to give similar details back to the team).
12. You move forward at an adrenaline loaded speed with your current direction, missing further details that were available from the team (use of combat speed in lieu of detail analysis mode).
13. By this point, your partner informs you that your severe shaking has created more damage than you have repaired (loss of fine and now gross motor skills).

If you want to do it right:

14. *Now* if you have read everything in this book up to this point and suddenly remember some of these skills, you finally step back to take things in after packing the wound "to let anesthesia catch up."
15. You see five suction canisters full and piles of blood soaked sponges.
16. The circulator is now gone to perform the seventeen tasks you asked them to do (you did not manage resources well and gave non-specific orders).
17. You start to take out the packs when in your subconscious you remember you need to *D.E.C.I.D.E.* what to do next so you step back and ask someone to find the circulator and more help.
18. You finally explain what is going on to anesthesia and obtain feedback from the scrub tech and the circulator as well as the patient's primary treating team.
19. You quickly learn valuable information from the team you were not aware of because it was not loaded to you in a manner you could use to correlate and besides that you already had a preconceived notion of what you believed was going on.
20. Finally, after obtaining the right information and writing the details out for everyone to see, the team develops several options on where to proceed.
21. By this time you have aborted the original plan for simpler plans that hopefully will get your patient out of the O.R. alive.

22. You decide on what appears to be the best option and a way out if that is the wrong one.
23. You remind everyone that you need to assess the success at a specific time interval.
24. You then proceed after giving very specific instructions to everyone and they have all repeated back to you exactly what was to occur.
25. You now move back to the table, your tremors gone and less stressed that you were five minutes previously.

Debriefing—After the Dust Settles

A key component to remember is that as quickly after the dust has settled and the crisis is over, the team must sit together and go through a debriefing to review the positive and negative aspects of the case. The debriefing is the most vital step which precedes the investigational team that will follow. Facts tend to be twisted and vary as time progresses and an individual's impression and responses will be clearer immediately after the incident than it is after time inputs thoughts from others. This makes it more difficult to understand what the participants were thinking during the incident and difficult to make changes to prevent the accident from occurring in the future. Once the retrospective nature of a subsequent investigation takes over, it is more difficult to know exactly what definitively was going on when the incident occurred. [142]

In a commentary on debriefings by Gen. Stephen R. Lorenz, Commander, Air Education and Training Command, he noted that in the debrief everyone makes a comment regardless if it is positive or negative. Knowing all we know from the science explained above, we all have our blind spots and can benefit from another's perspective. We must have faith in our team cohorts to be honest and forthcoming to assure we don't re-create failures because a team member was too afraid to speak up regardless of "rank." If the debriefing is held in a respectful manner the outcome should benefit the organization. [143]

Debrief Checklist

The team should address the following questions during a debrief:

- Communication clear?
- Roles and responsibilities understood?
- Situation awareness maintained?
- Workload distribution equitable?
- Task assistance requested or offered?
- Were errors made or avoided?
- Availability of resources?
- What went well?
- What should change?
- What should improve?

Figure 43 Simple Debriefing checklist
Adapted from *TeamSTEPPS* [144]

Preparation: "Are We There Yet?"

Gaba and colleagues have written what essentially has become the "bible" for anesthesia providers regarding preparation for crisis management. *Crisis Management for Anesthesiology* (1994), acknowledges that the field of Anesthesia is an event-driven, complex, tightly-coupled, very uncertain, and risky occupation. The field of Anesthesia has done an excellent job at delineating the crucial aspects of preparation for potential crises in their domain. The facets described above on origination of crisis from human error or other causes, the role of the system in latent conditions and predisposing factors, and how providers think in general and their shifts during a crisis are well outlined in their book.

To adequately prepare one's team, a team leader must understand how a problem or error can develop into an adverse outcome or worse, a disaster (crisis). One also needs to remember that not all disasters are internal and outside forces could shape the events inside the O.R. Observational vigilance, constant verification, and re-verification, environmental awareness (situational assessment), problem recognition, and prediction of "future states" are an important aspect of an anesthesiologist's daily workload.

To be prepared for this complexity, the field of Anesthesia teaches its field resource management to distribute tasks and workload over time and in consistency with resources, to prevent task competition or overload. In addition, they emphasize communication, inventory, and mobilization of available resources when needed, as well as continued monitoring and cross-checking of all data. All of this information has been cataloged into a reservoir of anesthesia crisis checklists which enable the team to rapidly move through known sequences, proven by time to yield the best outcome.

On top of these methods, the Anesthesia team is adept at preoperative planning including briefings involving the entire team if need be as well as generalized emergency preparedness. These concepts on team management have been instituted worldwide but acceptance and validation outside the field of anesthesia is lagging as noted previously. [7]

Unlike aviation and anesthesia fields, there is little to speak of in the surgical literature to determine how to best teach the teams to manage a crisis. It is not too difficult to find crisis intervention checklists for fires, explosions, and electrical accidents in the operating theater, with the goal to avoid and manage them by learning from the instructive cases. [145] Other checklists for other O.R. emergencies exist as well, but there is little to go by regarding managing the entire team through an O.R. disaster.

Gawande's group at Harvard did an initial study with small groups in 2011 revealing that groups followed known protocols more precisely if they used a checklist for different crisis scenarios as opposed to relying on memory. This was expanded to a much larger group and results published in 2013 confirmed that the use of a checklist decreases the missing of crucial steps in the management by the team. These studies did have limitations regarding the composition of the teams in that there were few actual surgeons involved in the simulation due to the difficulty in recruitment, but there were residents and surgery assistants.

While this is a major step in the right direction, as noted in these publications, these events are very rare with an average of 145 such events, including massive hemorrhage and arrest annually, for a hospital producing 10,000 procedures a year. With this knowledge, full team cooperation will need to be expected in future studies and protocols. [146-148] Unfortunately the majority of training in existence is focused on training the individuals how to manage scenarios but not the entire team.

My recommendation is that medical teams take the initiative to model their teams similar to aviation teams through the use of Team Training that is geared toward the operating room environment. Surgeons must keep in mind the ever-present stereotype currently held by our partners in the hospital regarding our ability to maintain leadership of our team during regular scenarios. To do this, we simply need to construct feasible simulation scenarios that do not disrupt large chunks of our facilities'

operating room times, to assure that everyone in the room trusts us. Once O.R. teams have mastered the ability to function as a cockpit in normal times to assure mistakes do not occur via faulty communication lines, then teams need to progress up a level to achieve the goal of functioning under duress and threat. Upon improving communication amongst the O.R. team, the team will become aware sooner when the projected path of an operation is being deviated from and can respond effectively. Similar to aviation and other high risk industries, every O.R. should keep posters on how to successfully conduct a team during a crisis. A team member could bring these into the room during the time of a crisis, not for the purpose of utilizing these as a checklist, but more as a quick reminder of how the team should conduct itself during these brief and vital periods of potential salvage of the situation. These same posters could be placed around the O.R. corridors to remind the staff of proper conduct during these rare events.

Aviator safety through cockpit management training was not accomplished by a single didactic session and teamwork icebreakers. This was only accomplished through:

- Focus on team training
- Simulation
- Interactive group debriefings
- Measurement and improvement of aircrew performance. [25]

Summary

At this juncture a surgical team reviewing the proceeding principles should be capable of the following:

1. Recognize how human error contributes to adverse events.
2. Understand how system deficiencies can allow a simple error to progress to a catastrophe.
3. Understand surgeons' cognitive functions during normal and abnormal circumstances.
4. Recognize that during a crisis there are pathways to success for the team and pathways to self-destruction based on the rapidity the team understands things are not normal and progress through the three stages above.
5. Remember that debriefing after any event is extremely vital for the team to improve.

With this knowledge teams and organizations may successfully reduce the risks during or after a crisis but unless they are truly a *resilient organization,* success may only be temporary. Resilience involves:

1. Ability to absorb a major blow and maintain function in the face of adversity.

2. Ability to bounce back extremely fast after an untoward event.
3. Ability to learn during the recovery phase and adopt productive practices to tolerate future occurrences (as noted previously, more rules do not usually help and frequently make matters worse).

The ability to absorb the blow immediately and maintain function is entirely dependent on the state of affairs of the organization prior to the event. If small quirks in the system seem to be bothersome and intolerable, instead of normal, in a complex system, a major adverse event will not be tolerated.

Complex systems are always prepared for small and large problems at all times and teams practice with the expectation that surprises will occur and learn to control these small events quickly they will learn to cope quickly with the unexpected, develop better communication pathways, develop swift feedback and learn to improvise comfortably. [88]

Your Own Worst Enemy: "Complacency kills, as do poor planning, carelessness, and bad judgment. While accidents do happen, we often have only ourselves to blame when we're in a pickle. Sometimes you have to learn from your own mistakes, but a wise man learns from the mistakes of others. If you fail to have a plan, you plan to fail."
Bear Grylls, Backpacker, October 2012,
http://www.backpacker.com/october-2012-danger-zones-escape-plans-you/survival/16946

Conclusion

Changing to a Resilient Culture in Any Health Care Organization

> "Managing Risk, should be a continuous and developing process that pervades our strategy. It must be integrated into our culture, our approach to problem solving and our decision making."
>
> ***Admiral Michael G Mulen*** 17th Chairman of the Joint Chiefs of Staff from October 2007 - September 2011; www.safetycenter.navy.mil.com

cul ture

a. the set of shared attitudes, values, goals, and practices that characterizes an institution or organization
b. the customary beliefs, social forms, and material traits of a racial, religious, or social group ; also : the characteristic features of everyday existence shared by people in a place or time
c. the pattern of human knowledge, belief, and behavior that depends upon the capacity for learning and transmitting knowledge to succeeding generations
d. the set of values, or social practices associated with a particular field, activity, or societal characteristic

From *Merriam-Webster's Collegiate® Dictionary, 11th Edition* ©2013 by Merriam-Webster, Inc. (www.Merriam-Webster.com)

Cultures: Some Are Pretty and Some Are Just Nasty!

Where do we go from here? Given the degree of difficulty hospitals are having in gaining trust in, and acceptance of O.R. time out checklists and medical team training, one would not recommend jumping in and developing a new checklist and hiring teams to train the staff without conducting appropriate staff interviews and gaining their input. As noted in CRM and MTT, without a culture change, no change will be possible.

> ...without a culture change, no change will be possible.

The definition of an *Organizational Culture* is very difficult to phrase precisely. Everyone knows what it is, but to describe it is difficult. Weick, Sutcliffe, and Reason describe it best as, "how the organization comes together with a similar outlook and prioritization, so they can achieve a collaborative goal." The vast amount of literature available to describe how to create a culture of safety in an organization and how to make a change in organizational culture surpasses the ability of this work.

As seen in Figure 44 the easiest way to summarize the requirements to establish a patient safety culture in any healthcare facility is that it predominately takes three major groups:

1. The organizational leadership
2. The physicians (surgeons)
3. The nursing and support staff

In non-health care organizations, leadership must have a) beliefs, b) values, and c) actions to support their unwavering advocacy of a safe environment. People must be continually informed of this value system through communications that are credible, consistent, and salient as well be provided with or offered a reward system that promotes safety (in lieu of punishing violations).

The perceived values and philosophy must be a) consistent, b) intense, and c) with consensus. Once the first two pillars are erected this will be followed by the erection of the third pillar: employee beliefs and attitudes, and behavior towards safety will become the norm. Everyone in health care truly believes in patient safety, therefore there is never a need to actually "change the organizational culture." No one working in a health care facility wants to admit patients to a facility where staff willfully engage in unsafe acts. The culture is already existent, but habits, norms, complacency, progressive regulation, competing interests between safety and production and cost saving commitments usually compete with these deep set values. [88]

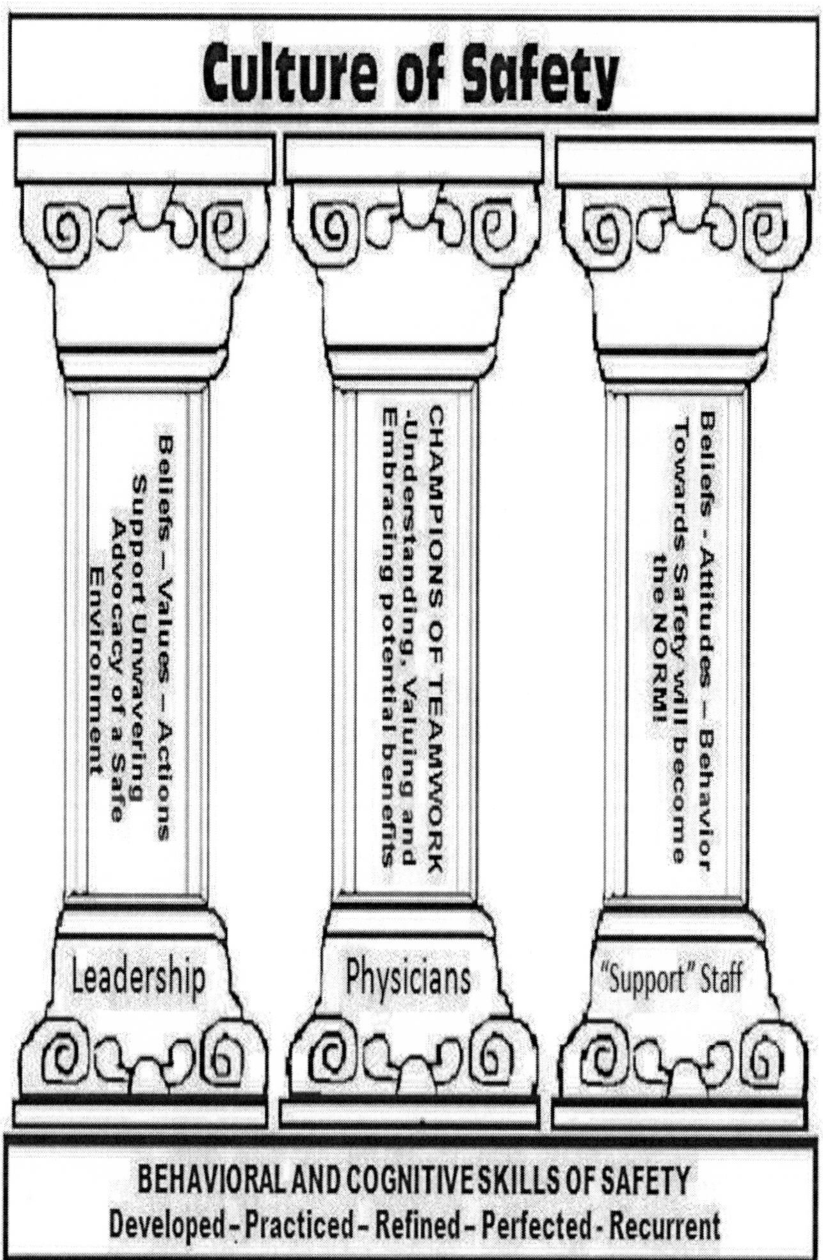
Culture of Safety
Beliefs – Values – Actions
Support Unwavering
Advocacy of a Safe
Environment
CHAMPIONS OF TEAMWORK
-Understanding, Valuing and
Embracing potential benefits
Beliefs - Attitudes – Behavior
Towards Safety will become
the NORM!
Leadership
Physicians
"Support" Staff
BEHAVIORAL AND COGNITIVE SKILLS OF SAFETY
Developed - Practiced - Refined - Perfected - Recurrent

Figure 44 Pillars of Patient Safety

A change in patient safety philosophy can only be brought about by a change in the healthcare facility patient safety culture. For a cultural change to occur, facility leadership, physicians and "support" staff need to have their priorities aligned.

Leadership must show that they have a) beliefs, b) values, and c) actions to support their unwavering advocacy of a safe environment.

They must assure that their values and philosophy toward patient safety are perceived by their employees as consistent, intense, and they have been accepted through consensus by all staff.

Facility employees must be continually informed of this value system through communications that are credible, consistent, and salient as well be provided with or offered a reward system that promotes safety (in lieu of punishing violations).

Physicians must support this philosophy verbally and by their actions in public, otherwise the remaining staff will not view this culture as being one designed by consensus. For this to occur, they must be actively involved in the construction of patient safety measures and monitoring.

Once the first two pillars are solidified, the support staff will understand that safety culture is the norm for everyone and employees' beliefs and attitudes, and behaviors towards safety will become the norm.

Figure 44 Pillars of Patient Safety

Adapted with permission from:

Reason J. *Managing the Risks of Organizational Accidents.* Burlington, VT: Ashgate; 1997. [53]

Weick KE, Sutcliffe KM, *Managing the Unexpected: Resilient Performance in an Age of Uncertainty.* San Francisco, CA: John Wiley; 2007. [88]

Salas E, Wilson KA, Murphy CE, King H, Baker D. What crew resource management training will not do for patient safety: unless…?. *J Patient Saf.* 2007;3(2):1-3. [150]

Culture of Safety: Surgeons as Leaders; "Big Deal! What's the Issue Here?"

As will be detailed in a moment, Salas pointed out years ago that unless physicians believe that teamwork is a focal point in the elimination of errors and adverse events, substantial universal change is unlikely. The catch phrase most often used in any conference concerning patient safety is: *buy in*, as in, "How are you going to get staff or leadership buy in?" It is certainly beyond the scope of this book to describe the volumes of literature on producing change and developing a culture of safety in its entirety but we will attempt to outline common concerns and potential solutions.

There seems to be five basic camps on patient safety beliefs amongst surgeons:

1. "Team Training and O.R. checklists have never been proven to provide substantial benefit." "We see these checklists as a waste of time, meant to empower

those who don't need to have role in the process. We want to see data to support these extra measures that show there is a safety benefit in terms of morbidity and mortality from safety checklists and Medical Team training. There are relatively few studies that reveal pertinent data to support this."

ANSWER: That's what the "top guns" used to say in the 80s, but studies have shown otherwise!

2. "We need leadership buy in to support the cause for heightened patient safety. Otherwise it is a waste of time." "Training of any type needs organizational leadership to run and maintain, not the surgeons."

   ANSWER: If we don't lead, who will?

3. "We are safe because we never have an O.R. crisis. These events rarely if ever happen!" "We haven't seen an adverse event here in forever."

   ANSWER: We should be prepared for anything that could pose a risk to our patients or staff that can have a significant chance of occurring and of lethal consequences if ignored.

4. "We are ready for anything. I am able to lead any team through any crisis without concern." "We don't need that. We have great teams. Before we had all these checklists we used to have the same team. Now we have different nurses, but we are still one team."

   ANSWER: That's not what our team partners say!

5. "We don't let O.R. disasters affect us. I am not personally at risk!"

   ANSWER: The Second Victim exists!

Myth #1: "Team Training and O.R. Checklists have Never Been Proven to Provide Substantial Benefit!"

Given the disparity in opinions on the need for effective methods to eliminate adverse events in patient care amongst physicians and surgical teams, it should be apparent that in an attempt to build an organization of "mindfulness," the best-intended mindful actions will be swept away by a force of individuals (or masses) who don't accept that there is enough documentation of success of these systematic changes. In a 2009 Interview, Pronovost says, "Safety should be a patient's right; if you are going to ask doctors to give up their autonomy and accept these standards, they have to be based on sound science and implemented wisely." [149]

To answer those who still question the need to make these suggested changes, one needs to assess what has happened in the transportation industry. While traveling was never unsafe for the majority of cases, incidents did happen that drew the attention of the media, TSA, and other transportation authorities. In 1991, the aviation industry was still debating the effectiveness of CRM as we are debating the effectiveness of MTT. Diehl summarized the quandary aviation safety experts faced at that early time in CRM, when he said:

> "In these times of tight budgets, management and government authorities can be expected to demand proof that preventive

> measures are in fact working. Here again, proving the effectiveness of human factors initiatives is very difficult, (e.g. crews can always comply with unpopular standard operating procedures during check-rides). Lastly, experts such as Dr. Clay Foushee (1987) have aptly noted that accidents, because of their relative infrequency, make poor scientific criteria. It is also axiomatic that proving the negative (accidents which were prevented) is even more difficult."
>
> "As noted above, oftentimes a priori scientific proof was unavailable. A proverbial '*Catch 22*' may have existed such as 'We can't use it until we know it works, and we'll never know it works until we try it.'" [27]

These statements were still circulating over ten years after the initial phases of CRM with much data to support its ongoing use. Keeping that in consideration, would any of us want to fly or travel in any public transportation knowing that there were significant communication gaps between the aircraft pilots, the rest of the crew, or the communication tower? In this day and age, with human factor and systems management training, the majority of near misses and tragic accidents are usually clear cut violations of CRM principles and persistent gaps in systems processes.

Telling surgeons that they must remain responsible while empowering others is as extremely difficult as training senior pilots to accept concerns from junior pilots. Yet, potentially many fatal scenarios could have been avoided if the team was able to voice concerns and draw attention to potential loose ends. Given that surgical teams are made of perfectionists who do not typically tolerate failure, it is difficult to understand the rationality of not wanting to spend three minutes to review a checklist, to assure the entire team is engaged and not just going through the bureaucratic motions sent down from above.

These steps have been shown to improve the working relationship of the team, reduce staff from having to leave the room, saving time and, more importantly, clearly eliminate much of the distraction that was mentioned above. In the end, patients and staff should feel safer and less stressed over potential mishaps. With this thought, a three-minute break prior to the incision really should not be a hardship.

Myth #2: "Training of Any Type Needs Organizational Leadership to Run and Maintain, Not the Surgeons!"

In Salas's commentary regarding CRM in medicine in 2007, he notes that CRM (MTT) is in wide use, yet if physicians do not believe that teamwork is critical in eliminating errors in medicine, it will be *"an uphill battle."*

Physicians must serve as champions through their understanding, valuing and embracing team training and its potential benefits. The attending in charge sets the tone for the entire health care team. Only through physician engagement will the entire team come together.

As seen in other high risk industries, unless patient safety concepts are ingrained in the physician culture, any training success will be short-lived. The partnership between the physicians, facility leadership and supporting services in making this a success is paramount for a lasting organizational vision of eliminating safety concerns at all levels. [150]

Tom Russell (Prior Executive Director of ACS) summarized it best in 2006 noting that good safety and teamwork climate are insufficient. "We blamed medical mistakes on the errant physician, the inadequately trained surgeon, or the negligent anesthesiologists." But at that time little attention was being paid to the effects of systemic problems. He noted that the study of human behavior showed that "people normally err, upon occasion, and that mistakes accompany natural reactions to latent, environmental factors." They "make mistakes when they feel the stress of interruptions, haste, fatigue, and lack of protocols. In the hospitals, long work hours, poorly maintained equipment, overstaffing, and inconsistent training of physicians… breed anger, anxiety, boredom and fear. These feelings interfere with our ability to concentrate. Individual limitations such as poor communications and interpersonal skills, memory problems, and personal issues also inhibit safe practice... the airlines now apply crew resource management technology which suggest simplifying procedures, standardizing process, and systematizing work by establishing protocols and guidelines." He reminded us that "...ultimately, it is the *surgeon* who is responsible for ensuring that the entire operative team delivers safe care. It is the surgeon who supervises and approves the series of events and supervises the handoffs that occur in hospitals when patients are undergoing major operations." [101]

In 2005, Wilson et al, noted that the organization alone cannot achieve a High Reliability Organizational (HRO) status without the integration of three key areas: organizational factors, team factors, and developmental strategies. That is, for the organization to succeed, the teams within the organization must also act in a high reliability fashion. An HRO committed to excellence actively seeks information to clarify what they don't know, designs reward systems recognizing the costs of failure and benefits of reliability, and communicates the concept of high reliability for safety to the entire organization. Collaboration and commitment to resilience among team members remains the mainstay for success. Team members serve as redundant systems to avoid, trap, and mitigate the consequences of errors. As Wilson states, "in order to prevent errors and ensure workplace safety, team members must do several things: a) ask for help when overloaded, b) monitor each other's performance to notice any performance decreases, and c) take an active role in assisting other team members who are in need of help. To accomplish this, high reliability teams demonstrate teamwork behaviors such as mutual performance monitoring, back-up behavior, and development of shared mental models."

These processes are not a one-time fix-all solution and the organization must monitor continuously to identify and correct non-routine/unsafe behaviors. "Team training needs to focus on teaching team members to identify errors and unsafe behaviors, provide constructive feedback, and correct any unsafe acts so that teams will be more effective during future events." Teams must be taught to perform these functions without further trainer intervention.

Organization level: Sensitivity to operations, commitment to resilience, deference to expertise, reluctance to simplify, preoccupation with failure.

Team level: Cross looped communication, information exchange, shared situation awareness, back-up behavior monitoring, shared mental models, assertiveness, collective orientation, expertise, adaptability, flexibility, planning, error management, feedback, and team self-correction.

Development strategies: Cross training, perceptual contrast training, team coordination training, team self-correction training, scenario-based training, guided error training. [151]

Myth #3: "We Are Ready for Anything. I am Able to Lead Any Team through Any Crisis without Concern because I am a Great Team Leader!"

As has been shown, surgeons tend to rate themselves very high on the "*I can manage a team effectively through a crisis*" and "*I am a great team leader*" totem pole. However, just as self-assessments are weak indicators of how an individual or team will respond to a crisis, self-assessments on teamwork depend on who you ask. [88]

Makary's 2006 study in 60 hospitals revealed that ratings of teamwork vary considerably depending on role. Overall, significant discrepancies were present in the perception of teamwork among physicians, anesthesia providers, and nurses. While surgeons and anesthesia providers rated teamwork the highest within their own discipline, teamwork ratings in their specialties were the lowest overall. O.R. nurses were given the highest ratings on teamwork, but rated surgeon teamwork at only 3.52 of 5.00. Surgeons rated teamwork among surgeons at 87% and anesthesia providers self-rated at 92.7%. It was acknowledged that nurses tend to communicate more "holistically" and physicians more succinctly. [152] In a 2007 Mayo Study by Wiegmann, it was shown that information conveyed in the operating room is often shared in a tense, ad hoc manner that is not conducive to comfortable communication. To make matters worse, 59% of non-physician respondents thought that surgeon attitudes and personalities negatively impacted teamwork. [85] While on the surface this may appear subtle, it would account for the disparity in interpretation in communication on approachability, ability to express concerns, and an overall culture of safety.

Provonst discussed the same discrepancy when reviewing data regarding impression of teamwork amongst ICU RNs and MDs, where MDs rated the RNs at a 90% rating for collaboration, but RNs rated the MDs at only 54%. [153]

In an interesting study by Helmriech's group, surveys were submitted to aviation and surgery teams. In their study, while pilots were least likely to deny the effects of fatigue on performance (26%), *70% of surgeons and 47% of anesthetists* denied the risks of those conditions. At the same time, while 97% of pilots and 94% of ICU staff rejected hierarchies where senior staff were not open to input from junior members, only 55% of surgeons believed junior staff should have input.

More disparaging was the discordance in the discernment of teamwork ability of surgeons whereby 73% of surgical residents, 64% of consultant surgeons, 39% of anesthesia consultants, 28% of surgical nurses, 25% of anesthetic nurses, and 10% of anesthetic residents felt the surgeons were team players.

The most frightening aspect of the study was that only 33% of hospital staff reported that errors are handled appropriately, 33% of intensive care staff did not acknowledge that they make errors, and over 50% of intensive care staff reported that they find it difficult to discuss mistakes. [154]

HAZARDOUS ATTITUDES

Attitudes that Impede Effective CRM

- Macho - "I can do it."
- Anti-Authority - "Don't tell me."
- Impulsivity - "Do something—quickly!"
- Resignation - "What's the use?"
- Missionitis - "Let's press on."

Myth #4: "We Are Safe because We Never Have an O.R. Crisis. These Events Rarely If Ever Happen."

Surgeons in the Operating Room need to adopt similar principles to that seen by many airline pilots. During the post-incident evaluation, the captain of the aircraft, whose prompt actions averted a catastrophe, stated it was the pilot's job to cope with the unexpected. "We have to anticipate the worst case scenario. We are not just up there to press a button and trust in the wonders of modern technology. We have to be ready for this eventuality." [53]

The medical industry is not at all unlike many others, where we retrospectively remember the desires we shared to do something to rid the organization of its potential for adverse events, but the same sentiment crops up frequently in the history of all organizational accidents: "*There always seemed to be something else more pressing.*" As adverse events become less common, the organization experiences a gradual deterioration of its defenses. During the periods of absence of any adverse events, the system has the impression that the safety system is operating effectively.

As an industry we must remember that safety is a dynamic non-event. That is, to assure safety happens, adverse events cannot occur. Constant change produces a stable outcome, not continued repetition of prior measures. Stability is achieved by assuring that changes in one system parameter are compensated by other parameters. "If eternal vigilance is the price of liberty, then chronic unease is the price of safety."

People who operate and manage high reliability organizations assume that each day will be a bad day and prepare for that. Like many complex organizations, health care safety cultures vary considerably, from pathological (don't want to know about safety issues, whistle-blowers are shot, failure is punished or concealed), to bureaucratic (responsibility is compartmentalized, failures lead to local repairs, new ideas present *problems*), and finally to generative (messengers are trained and rewarded, responsibility is shared, failures lead to reform, ideas welcomed). [53]

There is no such thing as absolute safety. As long as natural hazards, human fallibility, latent conditions and the possibility of chance exist, even the most intrinsically resistant organizations can still have accidents. *Lucky* but unsafe organizations can escape accidents for long periods of time. Effective safety management occurs when managers understand the forces acting on their organization and the types of information needed to fix their current position. The organization needs an internal *engine* to drive the organization in the right direction and the right *navigational aids* to plot their progress. The *engine* is fueled by motivation and resources. The organization must be fully committed and competent. Competency comes from knowledge and dissemination of information.

Commonly, managers attempt to direct control over incidents and accidents rather than regularly measure and improve processes known as potential risk factors for organizational accidents (design, hardware, training, procedures, maintenance, planning, budgeting, communication, etc.). Managerial goals should be focused towards maximal resistance to accidents, not zero accidents. Focusing on having zero accidents results in focusing too narrowly on negative events. [53] HRO's strive to assure that errors do not disable the organization, but do not focus on being error free. [88]

Myth #5: "We Don't Let O.R. Disasters Affect Us. I Am Not Personally at Risk!"

If these efforts fail, then surgeons need to be reminded of the "second victim." In the first section, it was clearly noted that distractions and stress in general predispose the surgeon or any member of the health care team, to a cognitive error. Having said that, one significant component not discussed above is the contribution that an adverse event has on creating more distractions for the surgeon and team members.

Perfectionism is an inherent trait of surgeons and other members of an operative team. Members of surgical teams are, by nature, almost uniformly pragmatic individuals who decisively perform invasive procedures that are designed to either improve individuals' lives, or are life-, sight-, or limb-saving. They display values that demonstrate "hero" qualities in the eyes of the majority of their patients.

In doing so there is always the expectation of a quick success. Furthermore, unlike other areas of medicine, the very nature of performing an invasive procedure links that action intimately to the patient's overall condition regardless of any true association. In this sense surgical teams are more accountable to their patients and peers in the expectation of a good outcome and failure is not tolerated by themselves or others. The obvious question to ask after any surgical failure is, "What did you do wrong?" [155] On top of that, unfortunately, most of us harbor maladaptive behavior in times of failure or significant change. During a 2008 survey of American College of Surgeons fellows, 8.9% reported committing a medical error within the preceding three months. The majority of these contributed this to a lapse in judgment, fatigue, lack of concentration, and other distractions. Further assessment of the responders noted that a prior medical error was independently predictive of high alcohol use and suicide ideations. While errors do occur outside the O.R., the consequences of an adverse event in the O.R. is more likely to be disastrous than in another setting, in the medical facility. Thus, anything that reduces errors reduces distractions from the surgical team and creates a safer environment for patients and staff.

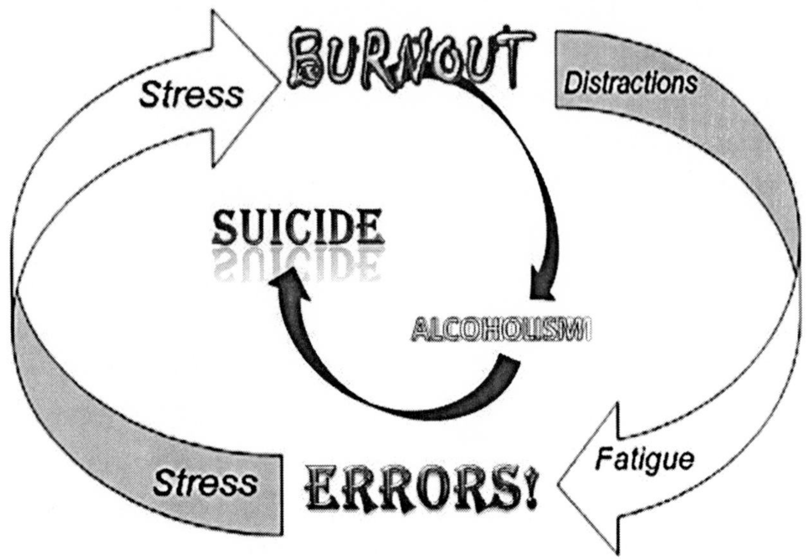

Figure 45 Relationship of errors on stress, fatigue, burnout, alcoholism, and suicide.
A recent American College of Surgeons Survey on burnout revealed a tight relationship between causing a patient error and stress, fatigue, burnout, alcoholism, and suicidal ideation. The only sure-fire way to cut the cycle is to reduce the stress induced by creating an error. [156-161]

Five Stages of Patient Safety Culture Maturity: A Systematic Approach to Risk Management: The MaPSAF Tool

In the end, it should be evident that in the field of medicine, just as in aviation and every other high risk industry, we should by this point understand where on the

Safety Culture ladder we want to rest. Dianne Parker and Darren Ashcroft coined a MaPSAF tool for a systematic approach to risk management, with a strong emphasis on multiple measures and targets into five stages.

The majority of systems begin at a very immature pathological level of interest in safety. As events occur in increasing frequency and damage, the institution becomes more aware of its role in preventing disasters due to human error or lack of training. Through leadership, system design, and teamwork the institution grows to a Generative Level at the top whereby safety is an ingrown mission centralized in the organization.

In their guidebook, *Crew Resource Management for the Fire Service* Randy Okray and Thomas Lubnau II describe the following FIVE IMPORTANT STEPS TOWARD CREATING A CULTURE OF SAFETY:

1. The organization must build trust among its members.
2. The organization must adopt a non-punitive policy towards error.
3. The organization must demonstrate a willingness to reduce errors in the system, which includes concrete steps towards error reduction.
4. The organization must provide training in error avoidance, detection, and management strategies.
5. The organization should provide training in evaluation and reinforcing error avoidance, detection,

and management. Debriefing should become the mainstay after all incidents.

Using other industries as an example, it should be clear that acceptance of these tools will never be an automatic process. Continued reinforcement of awareness behavior will be required until disaster prevention and CRM become a part of the routine. As seen in the Military, Aviation, Firefighters and other first responders, gaining appreciation for the vital importance of training in crisis management will be a long process met initially by denial but eventually with acceptance and appreciation. [27, 112]

Just as we expect safety to be a top concern for all staff involved in the preparation and flight of any plane we travel on, patients deserve to know that when they are in our O.R., if something unexpected happens, their team will be mentally and physically prepared to handle it. [162, 163]

The MaPSAF Tool

MATURITY LEVEL	APPROACH TO IMPROVING PATIENT SAFETY CULTURE
5. GENERATIVE	Creation and maintenance of safety culture central to organizational mission. Evaluation of effectiveness of interventions utilizing continued learning from success and failures to take meaningful action to improve.
4. PROACTIVE	Comprehensive approach towards promotion of a positive safety culture using evidence-based intervention across the organization.
3. CALCULATIVE	Processes limited to most recent very specific event
2. REACTIVE	Processes in response to latest disaster or recent regulatory review
1. PATHOLOGICAL	Shame and Blame Methods, Hide it!

Figure 46 Five Stages of Patient Safety Culture Maturity: Dianne Parker's and Darren Ashcroft's MaPSAF tool for a systematic approach to risk management, with a strong emphasis on multiple measures and targets into five stages. Systems tend to start off at a very immature pathological level and through leadership, system design, and teamwork grow to a Generative Level at the top whereby safety is an ingrown mission centralized in the organization.

Adapted with permission from:

Fleming M, Wentzell N. Patient safety culture improvement tool: development and guidelines for use. *Healthc Q*. 2008;11(3):10-15. [162]

Ashcroft DM, Morecrof C, Parker D, Noyce PR. Safety culture assessment in community pharmacy: development, face validity and feasibility of the Manchester Patients Safety Assessment Framework. *Qual Saf Health Care*. 2005;14(6):417-21. [163]

References

1 Dees RF. *Resilient Leaders: The Resilience Trilogy.* San Diego, CA: Creative Team Publishing; 2013.

2 Kolditz TA. *Extremis Leadership.* San Francisco, CA: Jossey-Bass; 2007.

3 Gazoni FM, Amato PE, Malik ZM, Durieu ME. The impact of perioperative catastrophes on anesthesiologists: results of a national survey. *Anesth Analg.* 2012;114(3):596–603.

4 Seeger MW, Sellnow TL, Ulmer RR. Communication, organization, and crisis. In: Rolff ME, ed. *Communication Yearbook.* Vol 21. Lexington, KY: U of Kentucky; 1998:231–275.

5 Venette SJ. *Risk Communication in a High Reliability Organization: APHIS PPQ's Inclusion of Risk in Decision Making.* Ann Arbor, MI: UMI Proquest Information and Learning; 2003.

6 Hermann CF. Some consequences of crisis which limit the viability of organizations. *Admin Sci Q.* 1963;8(1):61-62.

7 Gaba DM, Fish KJ, Howard SK. *Crisis Management in Anesthesiology.* New York, NY: Churchill Livingstone; 1994.

8 Ellison P. The 34th Rovenstine Lecture: 40 years behind the mask: safety revisited. *Anesthesiol.* 1996;84(4):965-975.

9 Kohn LT, Corrigan JM, Donaldson MS. *To Err is Human: Building a Safer Health System.* Washington, D.C: National Academies Press; 1999.

10 Institute of Medicine, Committee on Quality Health Care in America. *Crossing the Quality Chasm: A New Health System for the 21st Century. Committee on Quality of Health Care in America.* Washington, D.C: National Academies Press; 2001.

11 Gawande A. When doctors make mistakes. *The New Yorker*. February 1, 1999:40-55. http://www.newyorker.com/archive/1999/02/01/1999_02_01_040_TNY_LIBRY_000017427. Accessed Dec 31, 2012.
12 Gawande A. *Complications: A Surgeon's Notes on an Imperfect Science*. New York, NY; Metropolitan Books; 2010.
13 Joint commission on accreditation of healthcare organizations: universal protocol for preventing wrong site, wrong procedure. *Perspectives on Patient Safety*. 2003;3:1-11.
14 Brennan TA, Leape LL, Laird MM, et al. Incidence of adverse effects and negligence in hospitalized patients : results of the Harvard Medical Practice Study I. *N Engl J Med*. 1991; 324:370-376.
15 Laird N, Lawthers AG, Localio AR, et al. The nature of adverse events in hospitalized patients: results of the Harvard Medical Practice Study II. *N Engl J Med*. 1991;324:377-384.
16 Leape LL. The preventability of medical injury. In: Bogner MS, ed. *Human Error in Medicine*. Hillsdale, NJ: Lawrence Erbium; 1994:13-25.
17 Leape LL. Institute of Medicine medical error figures are not exaggerated. *JAMA*. 2000;284(1):95-97.
18 Calland JF, Guerlain S, Adams RB, Tribble CG, Foley E, Chekan EG. A systems approach to surgical safety. *Surg Endosc*. 2002;16(6):1005-1014.
19 Mehtsun W, Ibrahim A, Diener-West M, Pronovost P, Makary M. Surgical Never Events in the United States. *Surgery*. April 2013;153(4):465-472. http://www.surgjournal.com/article/PIIS003960601200623X/abstract. Accessed December 31, 2012.
20 Simon J, Ngo Y, Khan S, Strogatz D. Surgical confusions in ophthalmology. *Arch Ophthalmol*. 2007;125(11):1515-1522.
21 Helmriech RL, Ashleigh CM, Wilhelm JA. Evolution of CRM training in commercial aviation. *Int J Aviati Psychol*. 1999;9(1):19-32.
22 Lee T, Harrison K. Assessing safety culture in nuclear power stations. *Saf Sci*. 2000;34(1–3):61–97.

23 Dörner D. *The Logic of Failure: Recognizing and Avoiding Error in Complex Situations*. Reading, MA: Perseus Books; 1996.

24 Pizzi L, Goldfarb NI, Nash DB, Crew resource management and its applications in medicine. In: Shojania KG, Duncan BW, McDonald KM, Wachter RM, Markowitz AJ eds. *Making Health Care Safer: A Critical Analysis of Patient Safety Practices: Evidence Reports/ Technology Assessments, No. 43*. Rockville, MD: Agency for Healthcare Research and Quality; 2001. http://www.ncbi.nlm.nih.gov/books/NBK26999. Accessed December 12, 2012.

25 Cooper GE, White MD, Lauber JK. Resource management on the flightdeck: proceedings of a NASA/ industry workshop. In: *NASA Conference Publication No. CP-2120*. San Francisco, CA: NASA - Ames Research Center; 1980.

26 FAA. *Human Factors Guide for Aviation Maintenance and Boeing Maintenance Error Decision Aid (MEDA) Users Guide*. http://www.hf.faa.gov/hfguide/07/07_methods.html. Accessed February 2, 2013.

27 Diehl, A. Does cockpit management training reduce aircrew error?. *ISASI Forum*. 1992;24(4). http://www.crm-devel.org/resources/paper/diehl.htm. Accessed February 10, 2013.

28 Dekker S. *Field Guide to Human Error Investigation*. Surrey, UK: Ashgate Press / TJ International Ltd; 2002.

29 Vincent C. *Patient safety*. Chichester, UK: Wiley-Blackwell; 2010.

30 Babcock W. Resuscitation during anesthesia. *Anesth Analg*. 1924;3:208-213.

31 Arora S, Sevdalis N, Nestel D, Tierney T, Woloshynowych M, Kneebone R. Managing intraoperative stress: what do surgeons want from a crisis training program. *Am J Surg*. 2009;197(4):537-543.

32 Runciman WB, Webb RK, Klepper ID, Lee R, Williamson JA, Barker L. The Australian incident monitoring study: crisis management: validation of an algorithm by analysis of 2000 incident reports. *Anaesthia Intensive Care*. 1993;21:579-592

33 Runciman WB, Merry AF. Crises in clinical care: an approach to management. *Qual Saf Health Care*. 2005;14(3):156-163.
34 Webb RK, Currie M, Morgan CA, et al. The Australian incident monitoring study: an analysis of 2000 incident reports. *Anaesthia and Intensive Care*. 1993;21:520-528.
35 Charuluxananan S, Punjasawadwong Y, Suraseranivongse S, et al. The Thai Anesthesia Incidents Study (THAI Study) of anesthetic outcomes: II. anesthetic profiles and adverse events. *J Med Assoc Thai*. 2005;88(suppl 7):S14-S29.
36 Forrest JB, Cahalan MK, Reheder K. Multicenter study of general anesthesia: II. results. *Anesthesiology*. 1990;72(2):262-268.
37 Cooper JB, Cullen DJ, Nemeskal R, et al. Effects of information feedback and pulse oximetry on the incidence of anesthesia complications. *Anesthesiology*. November 1987;67(5):686-694.
38 Cooper JB, Newbower RS, Long CD, McPeekB. Preventable anaesthesia mishaps: a study of human factors. *Anesthesiology*. 1978;49(6):399-406.
39 Dripps RD, Lamont A, Eckenhoff JE. The role of anesthesia in surgical mortality. *JAMA*. 1961;178(3):261-266.
40 Clifton BS, Hotten WIT. Deaths associated with anesthesia. *Br J Anaesth*. 1963;35:250-259.
41 Edwards G, Morton HJV, Pask EA, Wylie WD. Deaths associated with anesthesia: report on 1000 cases. *Anaesthesia*. 1956;11:194-220.
42 Ponton-carss A, Hutchison C, Violato C. Assessment of communication, professionalism, and surgical skills in an objective structured performance-related examination (OSPRE): a psychometric study. *Am J Surg*. October 2011;202(4):433-440.
43 Sakran J, Kaafani H, Mouawad N, Santry H. When things go wrong. *Bull Am Coll Surg*. 2011;96(8):13-15.
44 Chung RS, Ahmed N. The impact of minimally invasive surgery on residents' open operative experience: analysis of two decades of national data. *Ann Surg*. 2010;251(2):205-12.
45 Markelov A, Sakharpe A, Kohll H, Livert D. Local and national trends in general surgery residents' operative experience:

do work hour limitations negatively affect case volume in small community-based programs. *AmSurg.* 2011;77(12):1675-1680.

46 Feanny MA, Scott BG, Mattox KL, Hirschburg A. Impact of the 80-hour work week on resident emergency operative experience. *Am J Surg.* December 2005;190(6):947-949.

47 Jarman BT, Miller MR, Brown RS, et al. The 80-hour work week: will we have less-experienced graduating surgeons?. *Curr Surg.* 2004;61(6):612-615.

48 Eckert M, Cuadrado D, Steele S. The changing face of the general surgeons: national and local trends in resident operative experience. *Am J Surg.* May 2010;199(5):652-656.

49 Yeo H, Viola K, Berg D, Lin Z, et al. Attitudes, training experiences, and professional expectations of US general surgery residents: a national survey. *JAMA.* 2009;302(2):1301-1308.

50 Pugh CM, DaRosa DA, Bell RH. Residents' self-reporting learning needs for intraoperative knowledge: are we missing the bar?. *Am J Surg.* 2010;199(4):562-565.

51 Weingart SN, Wilson RM, Gibberd RW, Harrison B. Epidemiology of medical error. *BMJ* . 2000;320(7237):774–777.

52 Hayward R, Hofer T. Estimating hospital deaths due to medical errors: preventability is in the eye of the reviewer. *JAMA* 2001;286(4):415–20.

53 Reason J. *Managing the Risks of Organizational Accidents.* Burlington, VT: Ashgate; 1997.

54 Gorovitz S, MacIntyre A. Toward a theory of medical fallibility. *Hastings Cent Rep.* 1975;5(6):13-23.

55 Gawande A. *The Checklist Manifesto: How to Get Things Right.* New York, NY: Metropolitan Books; 2009.

56 Vincent C, Moorthy K, Sarker SK, Chang A, Darzi AW. Systems approach to surgical quality and safety. *Ann Surg.* 2004;239(4):475-482.

57 Fischer J. Editorial opinion: is damage to the common bile duct during laparoscopic cholecystectomy an inherent risk of the operation. *Am J Surg* 2009;197:829-832.

58 Way LW, Stewart L, Gantert W, et al. Causes and prevention of laparoscopic bile duct injuries: analysis of 252 cases from a human factors and cognitive psychological approach. *Ann Surg*. 2003;237(4):460-469.

59 Hassan I, Weyers P, Maschuw K, et al. Negative stress-coping strategies among novices in surgery correlate with poor virtual laparoscopic performance. *Br J Surg*. 2006;93(12):1554–1559.

60 Berguer R, Smith WD, Chung YH. Performing laparoscopic surgery is significantly more stressful for the surgeon than open surgery. *Surg Endosc*. October 2001;15(10):1204–1207.

61 Simons D, Chabris C. Gorillas in our midst: sustained inattentional blindness for dynamic events. *Perception*. 1999;28(9):1059-1074.

62 Kahneman D. *Thinking Fast and Slow*. New York, NY: Farrar, Straus and Giroux; 2011.

63 Rasmussen J. Human errors: a taxonomy for describing human malfunction in industrial installations. *Journal of Occupational Accidents*. 1982;4(2-4):311-333.

64 Reason J. Understanding adverse events: human factors. *Qual Health Care*. June 1995;4(2):80-89.

65 Reason J. *Human error*. New York, NY: Cambridge University Press; 1990.

66 Hastie R, Dawes RM. *Rational Choice in an Uncertain World, the Psychology of Judgment and Decision Making*. Thousand Oaks, CA: Sage Publications; 2001.

67 Hogarth RM. *Educating Intuition*. Chicago, IL: University Chicago Press; 2001.

68 Hoffman DD. *Visual Intelligence: How We Create What We See*. New York, NY: WW Norton and Co.; 1998.

69 Kanizsa, G. Margini quasi-percettivi in campi con stimolazione omogenea. *Rivista di Psicologia*. 1955;49(1):7–30.

70 Gonzales L. *Everyday Survival: Why Smart People Make Dumb Mistakes*. New York, NY: WW Norton; 2008.

71 Gonzales L. *Deep Survival: Who Lives, Who Dies and Why*. New York, NY: WW Norton; 2003.

72 Fisher, GH. Measuring ambiguity. *Am J Psychol*. 1967;80(4):541-557.

73 Peterson M. The ambiguity of mental images: insights regarding the structure of shape memory and its function in creativity. In: Russkos-Ewoldson B, Intens-Peterson MJ, Anderson RE eds. *Imagery, Creativity, and Discovery: A Cognitive Perspective.* Amsterdam, AN: Elsevier Sceince Publishers B.V.; 1993.

74 Fioratou E, Flin R. No simple fix for fixation errors: cognitive processes and their clinical applications. *Anaesthesia.* January 2010;65(1):61-69.

75 Bastone K. Professor rescue. *Backpacker.* August 2009;37(269,6):64-65.

76 Abelson M. The Manual: finding lost hikers. *Backpacker.* August 2010;38(278,6):45-46.

77 Ecenbarger W. Buckle up your seatbelt and behave. *Smithsonian.* April 2009;92. http://www.smithsonianmag.com/science-nature/Presence-of-Mind-Buckle-Up-And-Behave.html#ixzz2GqIy5YQa. Accessed December 31, 2012.

78 Howe S; When disaster strikes! 5 true survival stories. *Backpacker.* October 2008;36(262-8):49-53. http://www.backpacker.com/october_08_when_disaster_strikes_top_survival_stories/articles/12607. Accessed January 1, 2013.

79 Thompson M. A dozen ways to die. *Backpacker.* October 2006;34(244.6):70-78. http://www.backpacker.com/survival_guide_skills_a_dozen_ways_to_die/article/12228. Accessed January 1, 2013.

80 Sussman A. Outdoor risks: win the mental game. *Backpacker.* May 2009;37(267-4):52. http://www.backpacker.com/may_09_win_the_mental_game/skills/13081. Accessed Jan 1 2013.

81 Endsley, MR, Garland DJ. *Situation Awareness Analysis and Measurement.* Mahwah, NJ: Lawrence Erlbaum Associates; 2000.

82 BalchCM, ShanafeltTD, DyrbyeL, et al. Surgeon distress as calibrated by hours worked, and nights on call. *J Am Coll Surg.* November 2010;211(5):609-619.

83 Moorthy K, Munz Y, Dosis A, Bann S, Darzi A. The effect of stress-inducing conditions on the performance of a laparoscopic task. *Surg Endosc.* 2003;17(9):1481–1484.

84 Feuerbacher RL, Funk K, Spight D, Diggs B, Hunter J. Realistic distractions and interruptions that impair simulated surgical performance by novice surgeons. *Arch Surg.* 2012;147(11):1026-1030.

85 Wiegmann DA, ElBardissi AW, Dearani JA, Daly RC, Sundt TM Disruptions in surgical flow and their relationship to surgical errors: an exploratory investigation. *Surgery.* 2007;142(5):658-665.

86 Sharps MJ. *Processing Under Pressure: Stress, Memory and Decision-Making in Law Enforcement.* Flushing, NY: Looseleaf Law Publications; 2010

87 Siddle B. *Sharpening the Warriors Edge: The Psychology and Science of Training.* 10th ed. Belleville, IL: PPCT Research publications; 2008.

88 Weick KE, Sutcliffe KM, *Managing the Unexpected: Resilient Performance in an Age of Uncertainty.* San Fransisco, CA: John Wiley; 2007.

89 Dekker, S. *Patient Safety: A Human Factors Approach.* Boca Raton, FL: CRC Press; 2011.

90 Rochlin GI, LaPorte TR, Roberts KH. The self-designing high-reliability organization: aircraft carrier flight operation at sea. *Naval War College Review.* 1987;40:76-90.

91 Perrow C. *Normal Accidents: Living with High-Risk Technologies.* Princeton, NJ: Princeton Press; 1999.

92 Chen Q, Rosen AK, Cevasco M, Shin M, Itani KM, Borzecki AM. Detecting patient safety indicators: how valid is "foreign body left during procedure" in the Veterans Health Administration?. *J Am Coll Surg.* 2011;212:977-983.

93 Billings CE, Reynard WD. Human factors in aircraft incidents: results of a 7-year study. *Aviat Space Environ Med.* 1984;55(10):960-5.

94 Helmriech RL, Merritt AC, Wilhelm JA. Evolution of CRM training in commercial aviation. *Int Jnl of Aviation Psychol.* 1999;9(1):19-32.

95 Aircraft accident report: Colgan Air flight 3407 Clarence Center, NY Feb 12 2009. *National Transportation Safety Board.* February 2, 2010.
http://www.ntsb.gov/doclib/reports/2010/AAR1001.pdf.
Accessed February 2, 2013.

96 Aircraft accident report: USA flight 1549 Weehawken, NJ Jan 15 2009. *National Transportation Safety Board.* May 14, 2010.
http://www.ntsb.gov/doclib/reports/2010/aar1003.pdf.
Accessed February 2, 2013.

97 Grogan EL, Stiles RA, France DJ, et al. The impact of aviation-based teamwork training on the attitudes of health-care professionals. *J Am Coll Surg.* 2004;199(6):843-8

98 Foster D, AGawande A, Singer S, BerryW. Factors associated with effective implementation of a surgical safety checklist. *J Am Coll Surg.* 2010;211(3):S108.

99 Khuri S. Safety, quality and the national surgical quality improvement program. *Am Surg.* 2006;72(11):994-998.

100 Brennan TA, Gwande A, Thomas E, Studdert D. Accidental deaths, saved lives, and improved quality. *N Engl J Med.* 2005;353:1405-9.

101 Russell T, Jones RS. American college of surgeons remains committed to patient safety. *Am Surg.* 2006;72(11):1005-1009.

102 Neily J, Mills PD, Eldridge N, et al. Incorrect surgical procedures within and outside of the operating room. *Arch Surg.* 2009;144(11):1028-1034.

103 Kelz RR, Tran TT, Hosokawa P, et al. Time-of-day effects on surgical outcomes in the private sector: a retrospective cohort study. *J Am Coll Surg.* 2009;209:434-445.

104 Wolf FA, Way LW, Stewart L. The efficacy of medical team training: improved team performance and decreased operating room delays: a detailed analysis of 4863 cases. *Ann Surg.* 2010;252(3):477-83.

105 Neily J, Mills PD., Young-Xu Y, et al. Association between implementation of a medical team training program and surgical mortality. *JAMA.* 2010;304(15):1693-1700.

106 Meeks DW, Lally KP, Carrick MM, et al. Compliance with guidelines to prevent surgical site infections as simple as 1-2-3. *Am J Surgery*. 2011;201(1):76-83.
107 France DJ, Leming-Lee S, JacksonT, Feistritzer NR, Higgins MS. An observational analysis of surgical team compliance with perioperative safety practices after crew resource management training. *Am J Surg*. 2008;195(4):546-53.
108 Wolf FA, Way LW, Stewart L. The efficacy of medical team training: improved team performance and decreased operating room delays: a detailed analysis of 4863 cases: discussion. *Ann Surg*. 2010;252(3):483-485.
109 Neily J, Mills PD, Eldridge N, Carney BT, et al. Incorrect surgical procedures within and outside of the operating room: a follow-up report. *Arch Surg*. 2011;146(11):1235-1239.
110 Henrickson SE, Wadhera RK, ElBardissi AW, Wiegmann DA, Sundt TM. Development and pilot evaluation of a preoperative briefing protocol for cardiovascular surgery. *J Am Coll Surg*. 2009;208:1115-1123.
111 Helmreich RL, Merritt AC. *Culture at Work in Aviation and Medicine*. Aldershot, UK: Ashgate Press; 1998.
112 Okray R, Lubnau T. *Crew Resource Management for the Fire Service*. Tulsa, OK: PennWell Press; 2004.
113 Crew resource management: a positive change for the fire service. Fairfax, VA: International Association of Fire Chiefs. http://www.iafc.org/files/1SAFEhealthSHS/pubs_CRMmanual.pdf. Accessed February 18, 2013.
114 Chopra V, Bovill JG, Spierdjk J, Koornneef F. Reported significant observations during anesthesia: a prospective analysis over an 18 year period. *Br J Anaesth*. 1992;68:13-17.
115 Kumar MM, Fish KJ. Anaesthesia crisis resource management training: an intimidating concept, a rewarding experience. *Can J Anaesth*. 1996;43:430-434.
116 McDonald JS, Peterson S. Lethal errors in anesthesiology. *Anesthesiology*. 1985;63:A497.

117 Helmreich RL, Schaefer HG; Team performance in the operating room. In: Bogner MS ed. *Human Error in Medicine.* Hillside, NJ: Lawrence Erlbaum; 1994.
118 Wrong site surgery project. Joint Commission Center for Transforming Healthcare.
http://www.centerfortransforminghealthcare.org/UserFiles/file/CTH_Wrong_Site_Surgery_Project_6_24_11.pdf. Accessed Jan 1, 2013.
119 Lingard L, Espin S, Whyte S, et al. Communication failures in the operating room: an observational classification of recurrent types and effects. *Qual Saf Health Care*. 2004;13(5):3330-3334.
120 Wiegmann DA, Elbardissi AW, Dearani JA, Daly RC, Sundt TM III. Disruptions in surgical flow and their relationship to surgical errors: an exploratory investigation. *Surgery*. 2007;142:658-665.
121 Symons N, Almoudaris A, Nagpal K, Vincent C, Moorthy K. An observational study of the frequency, severity, and etiology of failures in postoperative care after major elective general surgery. *Ann Surg*. 2013;257(1):1–5.
122 Greenberg CC, Regenbogen SE, Studdert DM, et al. Patterns of communication breakdowns resulting in injury to surgical patients. *J Am Coll Surg*. 2007;204(4):533-40.
123 Coffey M, Thomson K, Tallett S, Matlow A. Pediatric residents' decision-making around disclosing and reporting adverse events: the importance of social context. *Acad Med.* October 2010;85(10):1619-1625.
124 Zohar D. Safety climate conceptual and measurement issues. In: Quick JC, Tetrickle LE eds. *Handbook of Occupational Health Psychology*. Washington, DC: American Psychological Association; 2003:123-142.
125 Haynes AB, Weiser TG, Berry WR, et al. A surgical safety checklist to reduce morbidity and mortality in a global population. *N Engl J Med*. 2009;360:491-499.
126 Fedarko K. Feeling gravity's pull: a pilgrim heads into blue john canyon to pin down the meaning of survival. *Backpacker*. October 2006; 34(244:8):23-29.

127 The survival list: 101 skills guaranteed to get you out of trouble fast. *Backpacker.* October 2006;34(244:8):45-53.
128 Wiggins-Dohlvik K, Stewart RM, Babbitt RJ, Gelfond J, Zarzabal LA, Willis RE. Surgeons' performance during critical situations: competence, confidence, and composure. *Am J Surg.* 2009;198(6):817-823.
129 Flanagan JC. The critical incident technique. *Psychol Bull.* 1954;51(4):327-358.
130 Moorthy K, Munz Y, Forrest D, et al. Surgical crisis management skills training and assessment: a simulation[corrected]-based approach to enhancing operating room performance. *Ann Surg.* 2006;244(1):139-147.
131 Pauley K, Flin R, Yule S, Youngson G. Surgeons intraoperative decision making and risk management. *Am J Surg.* 2011;202(4):375-381.
132 Cohen I. Improving time-critical decision making in life-threatening situations: observations and insights. *Decision Analysis.* 2008;5(2):100-110.
133 Ripley A. *The Unthinkable: Who Survives When Disaster Strikes and Why.* New York, NY: Three Rivers Press; 2000.
134 Jenkins M. Panic. There's a backcountry killer on the loose. *Backpacker.* December 2007;35(254:9):60-119.
135 Gonzales L. How to survive (almost) anything. *NG Adventure.* Aug 2007;9(6):44-51.
http://www.nationalgeographic.com/adventure/survival/skills/index.html. Accessed Jan 1 2013.
136 Siebert A. *The Survivor Personality.* New York, NY: Penguin Group; 2010.
137 Survive!: what to do when the you-know-what hits the fan. *Backpacker.* October 2010;38(280:8):71-90.
138 Stevenson J. Survive anywhere. *Backpacker.* October 2006;34(244:8):39-43.
139 Crew resource management refresher. United States Coast Guard. 2002.
http://www.uscg.mil/safety/docs/PPTs/CRM_Refresher2002.ppt. Accessed February 2, 2013.

140 Driver W, Benner L. D.E.C.I.D.E. for hazardous materials emergencies: presented papers vol II: fifth international symposium on the transport of dangerous goods by sea and inland waters. Federal Republic of Germany Hamburg Federal Ministry of Transport; April 1978:24-27.
http://ludwigbenner.org/arch1.htm. Accessed February 20, 2013.

141 Benner L. D.E.C.I.D.E. in hazardous materials emergencies. January 2005 www.bjr05.net/papers/aopa_ottawa.pdf Accessed February 20, 2013.

142 McGreevy JM, Otten TD. Briefing and debriefing in the operating room using fighter pilot crew resource management. *J Am Coll Surg*. 2007;205(1):169-176.

143 Lorenz SR. Lorenz on leadership: creating candor. Luke Air Force Base. Decmber 3, 2009.
http://www.luke.af.mil/news/story.asp?storyID=123141471. Accessed January 23, 2013.

144 TeamSTEPPS Pocket Guide - 06.136. The Department of Defense Patient Safety Program in collaboration with the Agency for Healthcare Research and Quality AHRQ. Revised March 2008 Version 06.1
http://teamstepps.ahrq.gov/abouttoolsmaterials.htm#TrainingMaterials Accessed March 1, 2013.

145 Nishiyama K, Komori M, Kodaka M, Tomizawa Y. Crisis in the operating room: fires, explosions and electrical accidents. *J Artif Organs*. September 2010;13(3):129-133.

146 Ziewacz JE, Arriaga AF, Bader AM, et al. Crisis checklists for the operating room: development and pilot testing. *J Am Coll Surg*. 2011;213(2):212-217.e10.

147 Arriaga AF, Bader AM, Wong JM, et al. Simulation based trial of surgical crisis checklists. *N Engl J Med*. 2013;368(3):246-253.

148 Charuluxananan S, Punjasawadwong Y, Suraseranivongse S, et al. The Thai Anesthesia Incidents Study (THAI Study) of anesthetic outcomes: II. anesthetic profiles and adverse events. *J Med Assoc Thai*. 2005;88:Suppl 7:S14-S29.

149 Szalavitz, M. Study: a simple surgery checklist saves lives. *Time*. Wednesday, January 14, 2009. http://content.time.com/time/health/article/0,8599,1871759,00.html#ixzz2L5QN8JIx. Accessed February 2, 2013.
150 Salas E, Wilson KA, Murphy CE, King H, Baker D. What crew resource management training will not do for patient safety: unless…?. *J Patient Saf.* 2007;3(2):1-3.
151 Wilson KA, Burke CS, Priest HA, Salas E. Promoting health care safety through training high reliability teams. *Qual Saf Health Care.* Aug 2005;14(4):303-309.
152 Makary MA, Sexton JB, Freischlag JA, et al. Operating room teamwork among physicians and nurses: teamwork in the eye of the beholder. *J Am Coll Surg.* 2006;202:746-752.
153 Pronovost P. Intensive care unit safety reporting system (ICUSRS). Reported in: *Safety and Medicine.* http://ocw.jhsph.edu/courses/patientsafety/PDFs/PS_lec4_Pronovost.pdf. Accessed February 12, 2013.
154 Sexton JB, Thomas EJ, Helmreich RL. Error, stress, and teamwork in medicine and aviation: cross sectional surveys. *BMJ.* March 2000;320(7237): 745–749.
155 Bosk CL. *Forgive and Remember: Managing Medical Failure.* 2nd ed. Chicago, IL: University of Chicago Press; 2003.
156 Oreskovich MR, Kaups KL, Balch CM, et al. Prevalence of alcohol use disorders among American surgeons. *Arch Surg.* 2012;147(2):168-174.
157 Shanafelt TD, Balch CM, Bechamps G, et al. Burnout and medical errors among American surgeons. *Ann Surg.* 2010;251(6):995-1000.
158 Shanafelt TD, Balch CM, Bechamps GJ, et al. Burnout and career satisfaction among American surgeons. *Ann Surg.* 2009;250(3):463-71.
159 Shanafelt TD, Balch CM, Dyrbye L, et al. Suicidal ideation among American surgeons. *Arch Surg.* 2011;146(1):54-62.
160 Shanafelt TD, Sloan J, Satele D. Why do surgeons consider leaving practice? *J Am Coll Surg.* 2011;212(3):421-422.

161 Campbell DA, Sonnad SS, Eckhauser FE, Miller G. Burnout among American surgeons. *Surgery*. 2001;130(4):696–705.

162 Fleming M, Wentzell N. Patient safety culture improvement tool: development and guidelines for use. *Healthc Q*. 2008;11(3):10-15.

163 Ashcroft DM, Morecrof C, Parker D, Noyce PR. Safety culture assessment in community pharmacy: development, face validity and feasibility of the Manchester Patients Safety Assessment Framework. *Qual Saf Health Care*. 2005;14(6):417-21.

Acknowledgements

With love to my wife, Katherine, and children, Genesis, Bradley, Jarrod, Rachelle, and John for their love, patience, encouragement, and inspiration through the years (and especially over the months while writing this book).

To my son, Bradley, for his crafting several of the free-hand sketches used in the book.

To my son, Jarrod, for his expertise in editorial skills I desperately needed.

To my daughter, Genesis, for her patient photography and editing skills.

Thanks to Jenny and Rebecca Alpaugh for their superb editing skills utilized in scrutinizing the draft with a fine-toothed comb.

Special thanks to Glen Aubrey of Creative Team Publishing for his patience through my stubbornness in transitioning from a medical journal writer to a writer of a book with widespread purpose. His willingness to teach and nurture me as an author has been immeasurable.

Thanks to Justin Aubrey for his patience during the cover and figure designs (and my redesign requests).

I appreciate Randy Beck's patience during the website design and his assistance with creation of business cards and promotional fliers.

In addition, I am in gratitude for the individuals listed below for their informative and encouraging conversations, phone calls, and emails leading me in the right direction towards completion of this book.

Brigetta D. Craft, RN, MSN, DNP, Contract Patient Safety Program Manager/TeamSTEPPS Healthcare Team Training, AFMOA/SGHQ, Lackland AFB, TX

Robert F Dees; Major General U.S. Army Retired; Author *Resilient Warriors*, *Resilient Leaders* and *Resilient Nations*

Dr. Gene Deisinger, Ph.D. Deputy Chief of Police and Director of Threat Management- Virginia Tech, Blackburg, Virginia

Dr. Alan Diehl Ph.D. Author "Air Safety Investigators: using science to save lives-- one crash at a time"

Gordon Dupont, Aviation Safety Expert, CEO System Safety Services

Dr. Mica R. Endsley, PhD, PE, Chief Scientist US Air Force Pentagon

Bob Figlock, Ph.D. Navy Post Graduate School; Advanced Survey Design, LLC, Monterey, CA

Darren P. Gibbs, Colonel, USAF; Chief, Readiness & Emergency Mgt Division (A7CX)

Gordon Graham; Graham Research Consultants; Long Beach, CA http://www.gordongraham.com/about.html

Laurence Gonzales, Author, "Deep Survival"

Billy Jackson; Detective, retired, Newport News, Virginia, Police Dept.

William L Johnson, retired CG Commander (O-5) Ardent Sentry / Vigilant Shield Lead Planner JS J7 Joint Training / Joint Exercise Division

Bob Hahn, Associate Director, School of Aviation Safety. Naval Aviation Schools Command

Robin L. Homolak RN; OR Manager VA Long Beach Medical Center

Dr. Anthony LaPorta MD, FACS Colonel Retired, US Army, Professor of Surgery, Rocky Vista University School of Medicine

Representative Thomas Lubanau II BS JD; Wyoming State Legislature; Retired Fire Service Wyoming; Author "Crew Resource Management For the Fire Service 2002"

CDR Mitch Morrison, PhD; Chief, Aviation Safety Division; COMDT (CG-1131); U.S. Coast Guard Headquarters

Dr. Chan W. Park, MD FAAEM; Director of Simulation Medicine; McGuire VA Medical Center

Dr. Douglas E. Paull, M.D. Director, Patient Safety Curriculum National Center for Patient Safety

Dr. Peter J. Pronovost, MD, PhD, FCCMSr. Vice President for Patient Safety and Quality,Director of the Armstrong Institute for Patient Safety and Quality, Johns Hopkins Medicine

Dr. Matthew Seeger PhD, Professor Dean of the College of Fine, Performing and Communication Arts and Professor of Communication, Wayne State University

Bruce Siddle; CEO Human Factor Research Group; Author *Sharpening the Warrior's Edge: The Psychology and Science of Training*

Dr. Mark W. Scerbo, Ph.D., FHFES; Professor, Human Factors; Department of Psychology; Old Dominion University

Dr. Mathew Sharps, Ph.D. Author of *Processing Under Pressure – Stress, Memory and Decision Making in Law Enforcement*

Michael Spinks, Aircraft Safety Systems Specialist, commentator on: www.Examiner.com

John Tippett, Deputy Chief of Operations, City of Charleston Fire Dept.

Dr. Steven Venette, Associate Professor University of Southern Mississippi, Speech Communication

David S. Wade, M.D., FACS, Chief Medical Officer, Federal Bureau of Investigation

Dr. Eric Wiebke, M.D. FACS, Chief Surgery VAMC Hampton

And in addition the following First year Residents at EVMS for bearing with me as I continuously altered my approach to teaching this subject to them:

Dr. Eva Dentcheva, MD First year Surgery Resident EVMS

Dr. Wesley Glick, MD First year Surgery Resident EVMS

Dr. Benjamin Smith, MD First year Surgery Resident EVMS

Dr. Robert Lyons, MD First year Surgery Resident EVMS

Dr. Patricia U. Teschke, MD First Year Resident EVMS

Permissions

Permission was granted for quoted items and adaptations from the following individuals (listed in chronological order):

Stephanie Wright, Permissions Editor; Merriam-Webster Inc.; Merriam-Webster.com; http://www.merriam-webster.com/ http://www.websters-online-dictionary.org/definition.

Bear Grylls, Discovery Channel '*Man Vs. Wild*' www.beargrylls.com.

Billy Jackson, Detective, retired, Newport News, Virginia, police dept.

Robert F Dees, Major General U.S. Army Retired; http://resiliencetrilogy.com.

Thomas A Kolditz through Sheik Safdar, Permissions Coordinator, John Wiley & Sons, Inc., 111 River Street, Hoboken, NJ 07030.

Dr. Matthew Seeger, Ph.D Professor Dean of the College of Fine, Performing and Communication Arts and Professor of Communication, Wayne State University.

Steven Venette, Associate Professor University of Southern Mississippi, Speech Communication, Institute of Medicine; 2101 Constitution Av., Washington, DC 20418.

Atul Gawande (WHO Director of the "Safe Surgery Saves Lives" Initiative in 2006 and Author of *The Checklist Manifesto*) Professor in the Department of Health Policy and Management Professor of Surgery, Harvard Medical School, General and Endocrine Surgeon, Brigham and Women's Hospital; Department of Health Policy and Management, 677 Huntington Avenue, Kresge Building Room 400, Boston, MA 02115 http://gawande.com/.

Sonal Arora, Clinical Lecturer—Imperial College, London.

Raphael Chung, MD, MBA, FACS.

Samuel Gorovitz, Professor of Philosophy, former Dean of Arts and Sciences, Syracuse University.

Terry R. Lee, Environmental Psychology and Policy Research Unit, School of Psychology, University of St. Andrews, St. Andrews, Fife KY16 9JU, UK; {Through: Malcolm Jeeves Emeritus Professor Malcolm Jeeves, C.B.E.,

F.Med.Sci., F.R.S.E., P.P.R.S.E. School of Psychology and Neuroscience , University of St. Andrews}.

Professor Charles A. Vincent, Faculty of Medicine, Department of Surgery & Cancer Imperial College, UK.

R. Berguer, Department of Surgery, University of California Davis, Sacramento, California and Surgical Service at Contra Costa Regional Medical Center, Martinez, California 94553, USA.

Simons & Chabris (1999) Professor Daniel J. Simons; http://www.dansimons.com; Professor, Department of Psychology and the Beckman Institute for Advanced Science and Technology, the University of Illinois. Co-Author of *The Invisible Gorilla* with Christopher Chabris 2010.

Laurence Gonzales, Author *Deep Survival* 3216 Otto Lane Evanston, IL 60201 www.laurencegonzales.com.

Dietrich Dörner, Professor Emeritus, General and Theoretical Psychology at the Institute of Theoretical Psychology at the Otto-Friedrich University in Bamberg, Germany.

Charles M. Balch, M.D., F.A.C.S., Professor of Surgery and Oncology and Dermatology Deputy Director, Johns Hopkins Institute for Clinical and Translational Research.

Robin L. Feuerbacher, PhD, Energy Systems Engineering Program Lead & Assistant Professor; Tykeson Endowed Faculty Scholar; OSU-Cascades 105A; http://www.osucascades.edu/robin-feuerbacher.

Weick and Sutcliff; Kathleen M. Sutcliffe; Gilbert and Ruth Whitaker, Professor of Business Administration, Professor of Management and Organizations, Stephen M. Ross School of Business, University of Michigan.

Jill Fredston, Author *Snowstruck: In the Grip of Avalanches* 2005, Harcourt, New York/Cindi Squire

Sidney Dekkar, Professor in the School of Humanities at Griffith University in Brisbane, Australia; www.SidneyDekkar.com.

James F Calland, MD, Assistant Professor of Surgery, University of Virginia Health System

Charles B. Perrow, Professor Emeritus, Sociology, Yale University, Professor Emeritus Sociology 493, College St, New Haven, CT 06511-8907.

Gordon Dupont, CEO System Safety Services 23100 Willett Ave., Richmond, BC Canada V6V 1G1; www.system-safety.com.

Laura Pizzi, Pharm D Professor, Jefferson School of Pharmacy

Joint Commission, http://www.jointcommission.org/.

Mr Nicholas Symons, MBChB, MSc, MRCS, Chairman, London Surgical Research Group, Surgical Registrar, North East Thames; Honorary Clinical Research Fellow, Centre for Patient Safety and Service Quality, Imperial College, London.

Bill Runciman, Professor, Patient Safety & Healthcare Human Factors, School of Psychology, Social Work & Social Policy, Sleep Research Centre, University of South Australia, Research Fellow – Australian Institute of Health Innovation – UNSW, Clinical Professor, Joanna Briggs Institute, Faculty Health Sciences, The University of Adelaide, President, Australian Patient Safety Foundation.

K. Pauley School of Psychology, University of Aberdeen, UK

Steven Yule, Ph.D., Assistant Professor of Surgery Institution Brigham and Women's Hospital Department Surgery Brigham and Women's Hospital SRATUS Ctr for Medical Simulation 75 Francis St Boston MA 02115.

Izack Cohen.

Amanda Ripley Author *The Unthinkable: Who Survives When Disaster Strikes and Why* http://www.amandaripley.com.

Matthew J. Sharps, Ph.D., DABPS, FACFEI Professor of Psychology (Cognitive Science) California State University, Research Consultant, Fresno Police Department, Author of *Processing Under Pressure – Stress, Memory and Decision Making in Law Enforcement*, Looseleaf Law Publications, Inc.

Bruce Siddle CEO/Managing Partner, Human Factor Research Group, Inc. Millstadt, IL.

David M. Gaba, M.D., Professor of Anesthesiology, Perioperative and Pain Medicine, Stanford University, Director VA/PA Sim Center.

Mark Light, IAFC, CEO and Executive Director & Christine A. Booth, Executive Assistant: International Association of Fire Chiefs.

John B. Tippett Jr., CFO, MIFire Deputy Chief of Operations City of Charleston Fire Department 46 ½ Wentworth Street Charleston, SC 29401.

Mica R. Endsley, Ph.D., PE Chief Scientist United States Air Force AF/ST (4E130) 1075 Air Force Pentagon Washington, DC 20330-1075
https://www.satechnologies.com/contact.

Eduardo Salas, Ph.D. Pegasus & Trustee Chair Professor Department of Psychology, Institute for Simulation & Training, University of Central Florida.

Dr. Alan Diehl, Ph.D. *Author Air Safety Investigators: Using Science to Save Lives – One Crash at a Time.*

Tom Russell, MD, FACS, Past Executive Director of ACS.

Peter J. Pronovost, MD, Ph.D., FCCMSr. Vice President, Patient Safety and Quality, Director of the Armstrong Institute for Patient Safety and Quality, Johns Hopkins Medicine.

Tait D. Shanafelt, MD Professor of Medicine Mayo Clinic.

Mark Fleming Ph.D., MSc, MA CN Professor of Safety Culture, Associate Professor Department of Psychology, Saint Mary's University.

Darren M Ashcroft BPharm MSc Ph.D., Professor of Pharmacoepidemiology, School of Pharmacy & Pharmaceutical Sciences, University of Manchester.

Representative Thomas Lubanau II BS JD.

About The Author

Kenneth A. Lipshy MD, FACS (Fellow American College of Surgeons) has been an active surgical leader in the Veterans Administration Health Care System. Prior to federal service he was in private practice for eight years. His private practice career was preceded by a three-year surgery oncology fellowship at Virginia Commonwealth University. His surgical education began during an internship at Ben Taub Hospital – Baylor College of Medicine Houston, TX and was followed by completion of his surgery residency at Marshall University Huntington, West Virginia.

His interest in surgical error and its relationship to crises was sparked during his training while serving in over two dozen medical centers during his career. However, his true interest flourished while serving as assistant scoutmaster in a local troop where he recognized a correlation between wilderness misadventures and O.R. disasters. This, combined with close associations with local members of all branches of the armed services as well as first responders, opened the door to a wealth of information on these topics as they relate to fields that are constantly at risk of facing crises.

Appendices

Appendix A

Heuristic Influence on Cognition

"Aoccdrnig to rscheearch, it deosn't mttaer in what oredr the ltteers in a word are sohwn, the olny iprmoatnt tihng is that the frist and lsat ltteer be in the rghit pclae. The Rset can be a taotl mese and you can still raed it wouthit a problem. This is bcuseae the huamn mnid desos not raed ervey lteter by istlef, but the word as a wlohe. Azanmig, huh? "
Figure 1 Positive Attributes of Heuristics: One <u>**Positive Attribute**</u> is that this process works quickly and relatively effectively. As one recalls learning to read as a child, it is clear we learn in a very s-e-q-u-e-n-t-i-a-l manner. We read each letter slowly till a word appears. This process is cumbersome and time consuming. As time progresses, we learn to read in a more automated (subconscious) format, frequently skipping letters to form whole words in our mind based on past experience with that sequence scenario. As one reads the words, the letters are purposefully placed close enough to their original context so that the human mind is capable of filling in the remainder to allow us to quickly read this otherwise illegible paragraph. If read in a slow sequential manner, word recognition would be less likely.

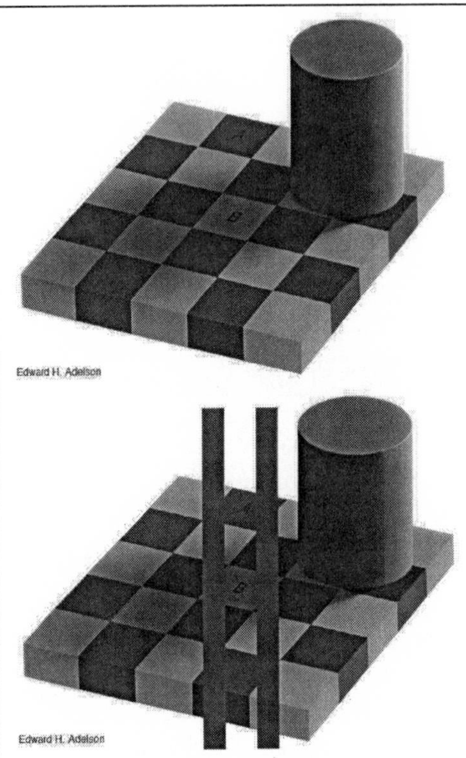

Figure 2 Checker Shadow:
Another excellent model is Edward Adelson's Checker Shadow experiment from 1995, shown above. Here a single white checkerboard square, that appears to be sitting in the middle of a shadow of a nearby cylinder, appears to be darker than a similar square located in an area that is not in the shadow. In actuality, these two squares are the same color (if you are still a disbeliever there is a convincing video at this website:

http://www.openculture.com/2011/08/mit_checker_shadow_illusion.html)

(Adelson E Checkershadow Experiment http://web.mit.edu/persci/people/adelson/checkershadow_downloads.html
Accessed Dec 31 2012)

http://web.mit.edu/persci/people/adelson/checkershadow_downloads.html accessed October 30 2012; ©1995, Edward H. Adelson.
"These checkershadow images may be reproduced and distributed freely"

Confirmation Bias and Fixation

Addendum Figure 3 Fixation Errors:

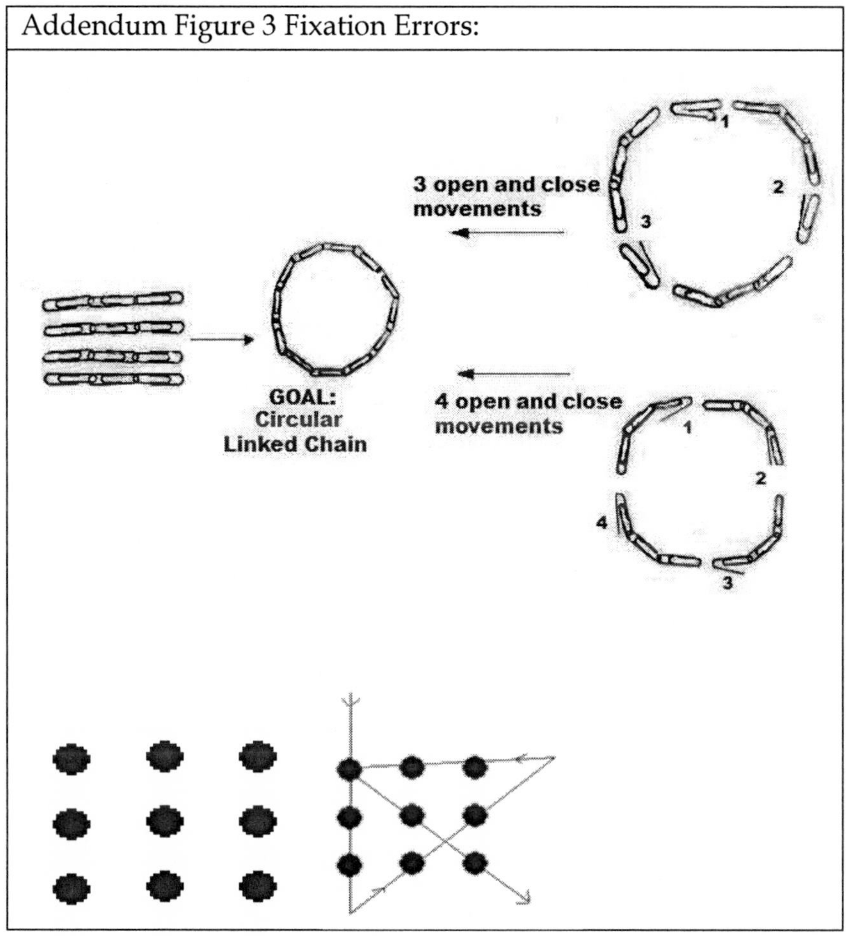

Fixation Error in the prevention of simple chain link and connect the dot problem solution

Adapted from Fioratou E, Flin R. No simple fix for fixation errors: cognitive processes and their clinical applications. Anaesthesia 2010; 65:61-69

As described on page 93, Fioratou's group designed an experiment tasking subjects to connect four strands composed of three paper clips joined together, into a circle, but allowed them to only use three open and closing movements (i.e. only three paper clips could be pulled apart and then closed). Ninety-seven percent of subjects could not do this. It turns out that the majority of subjects focused on the goal of joining paper clip strands and did not consider the option of taking one strand apart to use three separate clips to join the remaining three clips.

The same scenario is seen when one is asked to connect three rows of three dots with four straight lines without lifting the pencil. The mind attempts to force the solution to involve possibilities that only allow the lines to stay within the confines of the nine dots and does not typically allow one to consider going outside the box created by the nine lines. While these may seem like simple entertaining mind tests, it is also a keen reminder to us that we must be ready to accept an alternative maneuver that may be in a direction away from our goal, such as calling for a surgical airway when our goal is to intubate the patient with an endotracheal tube.

Appendix B

System's Role in Error Mitigation

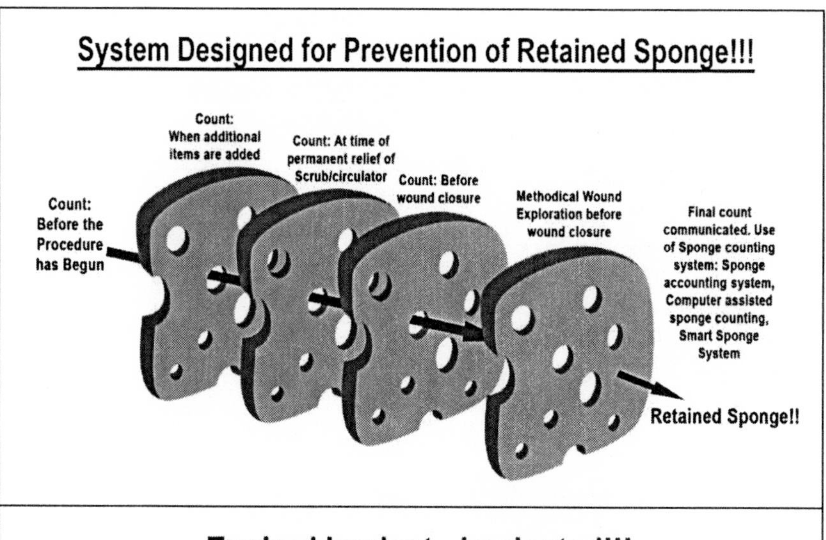

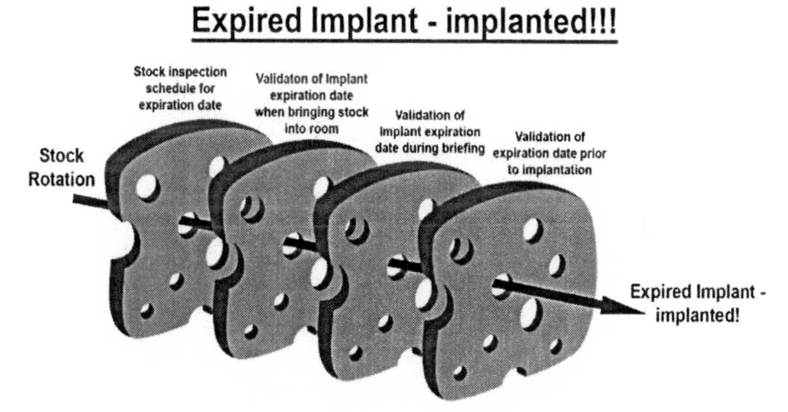

Figure 5 System Safety Nets and Subsequent Failures in the evolution of two well-known surgical adverse events:
a) Retained Surgical Item, and b) Implantation of Expired Implant

Report by Diehl on Accident Reduction in Multiple Aviation Industries in Multiple Aircraft Types in the 1980s

Kind of Operation	Procedural "Slips"	Perceptual Motor "Bungles"	Decisional "Mistakes"
General Aviation	5%	44%	52%
Airlines	19%	25%	56%
Military	11%	37%	53%

Organization/Subjects	Materials	Accident Rates
Bell Helicopters, Inc. Worldwide, Jetranger Pilots	ADM	36% Decrease
Bell Helicopters, Inc. U.S. Only, Jetranger Pilots	ADM	48% Decrease
Petroleum Helicopters, Inc. Commercial Pilots	ADM & CRM	54% Decrease
U.S. Navy All Helicopters, Crewmembers	CRM	28% Decrease
U.S. Navy A-6 Intruder, Crewmembers	CRM	81% Decrease
U.S. Air Force MAC Transports, Crewmembers	CRM	51% Decrease

One decade after United Airlines developed their Crew Resource Management training program, Alan Diehl, a world renowned aviation safety investigator, presented a seminar at the International Society of Air Safety investigators. Surprisingly, after 10 years, it appears there was still ongoing debate regarding the effectiveness of CRM. In his report, Diehl reviewed the results of 28 NTSB reviewed accidents and 169 US Air force accidents from1987-89. His conclusion was that 24 of the 28 NTSB and 113-169 US Air Force accidents involved aircrew error (Details seen in figure below). After thorough review of these accidents and existing CRM training he detailed the needs for an effective Cockpit management training program as:

1. Attention management issues include understanding how distractions and "error chains" can be avoided.
2. Crew management issues teach the importance of proper communications, division of responsibilities, leadership, and teamwork.
3. Stress management concepts focus on understanding the effects of life stress events as well as providing in-flight stress coping strategies.
4. Attitude management concepts describe the methods of recognizing and controlling certain hazardous attitudes and behavioral styles.
5. Risk management issues focus on the rational evaluation of qualitative and quantitative information related to operational hazards.

In his review of the results of Aeronautical decision Making (ADM) or CRM programs Diehl found an error reduction rate of 8-46% and accident reduction success rate of 28-81%.

Diehl, A. Does cockpit management training reduce aircrew error; *ISASI forum,* 1992; 24(4) available at: http://www.crm-devel.org/resources/paper/diehl.htm

Index

A

B

C

D

E

F

H

I

J

K

L

M

N

O

P

R

S

T

U

V

W

CPSIA information can be obtained
at www.ICGtesting.com
Printed in the USA
FFOW05n2206040214

9 780989 797542